They Didn't Teach Us THAT In Dental School

Strategies for Dental Practice Success

By Dr. Steven M. Katz

First published by Dog Ear Publishing
4010 W. 86th Street, Ste H
Indianapolis, IN 46268
www.dogearpublishing.net

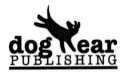

ISBN: 978-1-4575-2811-8

This book is printed on acid-free paper.

Printed in the United States of America

"Dr. Steven Katz is one of the top coaches in dentistry. As a practice owner and clinician he has seen it all - tragedy, failure, and eventually tremendous success. Steve's compassion and desire to help others combined with his highly productive practice make him the perfect person to motivate his colleagues. In 'They Didn't Teach Us _THAT_ In Dental School' Dr. Katz reveals all of the tips, tricks and secrets you need to know to achieve similar success. We congratulate him on the publication of this meaningful and fantastic book!"

—Dr. Richard Madow
The Madow Brothers

"The title, "They Didn't Teach Us _THAT_ In Dental School is a great synopsis of its contents. This well written and easy to read book is a wonderful guide to the "THAT" which is the measure of the success of your practice, and the "THAT" which goes into building and maintaining it.

As Dr. Katz explains, "helping dentists and their teams realize the full potential of their practices and how to enjoy the success of realizing that potential", is the intent of this informative book. You can enjoy the contents, but you will benefit by applying its wisdom to your professional life.

—Mark Marinbach
Founder of Nu-Life Restorations of Long Island

"Dr Katz has hit a home run in his first time at bat. This book is a very practical guide to dental practice success, focusing on what can be done, not what can't be done.

Leadership, development, verbal and clinical skills, empowerment of your team, computer utilization, communication skills, and much, much more are discussed. In a clear, simple and fun manner, Dr Katz has given the dental team a "bible" on how to enjoy dentistry, and be successful at it. This is a MUST read for the novice or seasoned professional.

I congratulate Dr Katz for putting together this truly amazing book. It is the most exciting read in dentistry I've come across in the past 30 years."

—Fred Danziger DDS, FAGD, FACD
Charleston, SC

"They Didn't Teach Us <u>THAT</u> in Dental School" is the secret sauce that separates the truly awesome from the average. Dr. Katz succinctly provides the information needed to help take your practice to the next level. Having known Dr. Katz for over a decade, I can tell you he absolutely is the real deal! He "Walks the Walk as well as Talks the Talk" bringing an unwaveringly positive attitude to all aspects of life and a true passion for systems that work in the real world. I have enjoyed watching many of his "students" benefit from his principles and concepts, increasing organization, enjoyment, and revenue."

—Scott Sanford
Founder of HealthyIT, A Computer Service and Support Company

Dedication

*This book is dedicated
to the memory
of my wonderful friend,
Mitch Cutler.*

It is said that in order to live a fulfilling life you need to fill each day with learning something, helping someone and exhausting the full range of emotions from tears to laughter. If this is true, then anyone who ever knew Mitch derived fulfillment from their relationship with him. I was fortunate to be able to call Mitch a dear, dear friend for 3 decades. For me he was a source of knowledge and inspiration, someone who helped me through difficult times in my life, a dear friend with whom I shared many laughs and recounts of family adventures. When he passed away in mid-2012 I shed many tears, BUT these tears were not because Mitch was gone, but instead they were for the joy that our relationship brought me throughout the 30 years that we were friends.

Tears are sometimes an inappropriate response to death. When a life has been lived with complete honesty, complete compassion, complete generosity, complete loyalty and complete joy, then the correct response to death's punctuation mark is a smile. Smile with me as I write about my friend Mitch.

For most of my years in practice, Mitch was my Henry Schein Sales Representative. He taught me the importance of true relationships in the business world. He taught me about trust and a deep concern for others. This is how Mitch became such an amazingly successful sales person. I always knew with Mitch that the relationship and helping me was what mattered most to him, and it was because of this that I never asked anyone else when I needed something for my practice. His relationship with his clients was more about showing how much he cared.

I will never forget how Mitch responded when I introduced him to Walter Hailey and Boot Camp, down in Texas in 1994. He enjoyed that experience so much that I thought he was going to develop a southern drawl. I always loved Mitch's thirst for learning and how he embraced new ideas. Even more impressive was how he shared everything he learned with others. Mitch shared the lessons of the Boot Camp experience with every dental professional he has ever known.

Mitch was always there for me. When I virtually lost my practice and I became deeply depressed as a result of a series of life tragedies 10-12 years ago, no one helped me more in getting me back on my feet. He called every single day and listened to me describe my concerns. Then he encouraged me and stood beside me as small strides lengthened and he became a driving force to the success I have achieved since that time. When I stopped working for the NY Jets, he encouraged me to take on a new challenge and he repeatedly encouraged me to become a "Consultant" and teach other dentists about recovery. The success I am enjoying in working with other dentists today is because of how Mitch motivated and encouraged me.

Perhaps the most memorable experience I ever had with Mitch occurred the day before he went to Mexico for treatment of his cancer 2 years before he ultimately passed. That day he had arranged a round of golf for the two of us and two other dental colleagues. Three of us WERE golfers and Mitch wanted to play. Well, to everyone's surprise, especially Mitch, that day he caromed shots off golf carts and rocks, he ricocheted shots off trees and he soundly beat all of us. Some of the shots he pulled out of his bag that day will never be duplicated, but that's because Mitch was an original. I never spent a day with Mitch where he did not have a huge smile on his face, but that day was the most joyful I had ever seen him. He couldn't wait to play again. Unfortunately, we never had the opportunity to play another round together, but I can say that every time I play golf now, wherever I play and whoever I'm playing with, I have Mitch sitting right beside me in the golf cart and I always have a fun time thinking about him.

Over the 6 years that Mitch battled cancer he taught all of us the true meaning of courage. It was truly remarkable how positive he was with all that he was enduring; yet Mitch always had the biggest smile in the room. My entire team welcomed his visits with his warm greeting, his hugs for everyone and his insistence that everything was "Good! Good! Good!". No matter what was going on, Mitch's presence always improved the lives of everyone he came in contact with. He is the most inspiring person I have ever known.

Even in his last days, Mitch was able to make a major impact on my life. Just a few weeks before he passed Mitch called me and asked me to deliver a tribute/eulogy at his looming "Celebration of Life". A few days later I spent some time with him, sitting on his bed, reliving some of our mutual experiences. I told him that I was beginning to compose his eulogy. He looked at me and said he wanted to read it. When I left his house, with its magnificent view of the Croton reservoir that afternoon, I was deeply inspired. I stopped right around the corner from the house at a burger joint and wrote my thoughts in a very short time. That is when it struck me how brilliant Mitch was. He was giving me the opportunity to tell him what I thought about him and how he had affected me while he was still alive. What could be better? Everyone should have that opportunity to honor their loved ones before it is too late. One week later I sat on his bed with him again while he read what I had written. He turned to me, hugged me, and gave me that huge Mitch smile and told me he was proud of how he had affected me. It was one of the most wonderful moments of my life. He taught me a great lesson in this exercise. We must express to all of our loved ones what they mean to us each and every day. Take time daily to hug and love your spouse or significant other, your children and express your love to those who affect you every day of your life.

Life comes without guarantees... except that laughing will brighten your day, smiling will enhance your eyes and having true friends will change your life.

If I were to ask you to name:

- The 5 wealthiest people in the world...or

- The last 5 Academy Award winners for best actor and actress...or

- Ten people who have won a Nobel Prize...

How would you do?

The point is that none of us remember the headliners of yesterday. These are individuals who have achieved incredible things. But, the applause dies, certificates fade and awards tarnish.

Now if I ask you to:

- Name 3 friends who helped you through a difficult time...or

- Recall 3 people who made you feel special and appreciated...or

- List 3 people who you enjoy spending time with, isn't that easier?

The lesson is that the people who make a difference in your life are not the ones with the most credentials, the most money or the most awards. They are the ones that care the most. And no one cared about people more than Mitch. Mitch for this I miss you.... but your spirit lives on for me in what I do on a daily basis and in the writing of this book.

Table of Contents

Section One:
What They Taught Us In Dental School About How to Manage a Dental Practice   9

Section Two:
They Didn't Teach Us THAT in Dental School   15

Category One:
Leadership   17

Category Two:
Business Prowess

Category Three:
People

Category Four:
Sales

Section Three:
The 15 Most Frequently Asked Questions
& Other Scripts   169

Section Four:
I Appreciate You's !   227

Section Five:
About the Author   231

Section Six:
About Smile Potential   233

Foreword
By Kirk Behrendt

It was March of 2007, and I was early in my speaking career giving a lecture to the Peninsula Hospital Dental Society on Long Island. I remember really sweating this group. Everyone had warned me. These guys had a reputation of being VERY tough — some of them even ruthless.

I can remember how nervous I was that day. My hands were sweating and I was hugely sleep-deprived from the night before. Somehow, I managed to get to the first break without getting eaten alive. As I was coming back from the restroom, a really nice dentist stopped me to give me some very kind words. I'll never forget his face. I remember his quiet confidence, his smile and his presence. I don't remember exactly what he said, but whatever it was, it was the perfect boost that I needed. His words brought a renewed energy and confidence to me. For the rest of the day, I anchored in on his smile from the audience. No matter where I looked in the large and daunting room, coming back to his face, gave me the safety I needed to carry on.

That man was Dr. Steve Katz.

And that is the best way to describe him. In the midst of uncertainty, anxiety and pure stress, he has an uncanny way to make you feel at peace. He serves as a guiding light to everyone in his path. It is no accident this dentist from Malverne, Long Island has created such a successful dental practice that has changed so many lives.

Dentistry is truly the most amazing profession if it is practiced the right way. The key is finding what is truly the "right way" for you. Every so often you come across mentors and Sherpas whom offer great advice from the road ahead. As humans, we have a choice to listen to this advice, gain from their help, and make our journey less painful. The other choice we have is to continue the climb while attempting to navigate the path by ourselves.

What you are about to read will greatly improve your life if you let it. Dr. Katz has spent a lifetime gathering the "secrets" of how to create a successful dental practice. Many of the answers to the redundant questions dentists and team members get every day are revealed in this book. Not only does he reveal the answers to these critical questions but more importantly, he greatly articulates the understanding behind WHY patients ask these questions and WHY the answers work. Learning more about the WHY itself, is a lifetime of intentional work.

I have always said that there are two types of practices in dentistry: People who fix teeth and people who change lives. They are two completely different businesses. Neither is good or bad. You just have to pick what you want to experience yourself in this great profession.

If you choose to change people's lives you will need

some help along the way, some perspective, some wisdom. My challenge is to let the words of these pages affect you, guide you, and lift you in the years to come. May they give you the quiet confidence, smile and presence to help those you meet on your path that may feel a little nervous or uncertain at times. When you do, it will change their lives, as well. Just like Dr. Steve Katz did for me, and has done for so many others in this world.

I wish you a very successful future in this great profession.

—Kirk Behrendt
March 2014

Kirk Behrendt is the founder and CEO of Act Dental. He is a renowned dental practice coach, international speaker and author. He is a rousing speaker who receives numerous standing ovations at his presentations. Peter Dawson called him "The best motivator I have ever heard."

Kirk has competed internationally in 4 Ironman Triathlons. He loves cycling, basketball, stand-up comedy, and most of all, spending time with his wife, Sarah, and children Kinzie, Lily, Zoe & Bo.

Introduction

The basic premise of this book is that all of us who entered dentistry as a profession were underprepared in Dental School for the realization that dentistry is a business. We were taught virtually no business principles that could be applied to the management of our eventual practices. We were taught very little about the "people skills" necessary to develop success in the environment of a dental practice. We were prepared for the clinical challenges we would face, to the best that could be accomplished in the context of "minimum requirements for graduation". Some programs were obviously stronger than others, but all seemed to lay a sufficient groundwork for the clinical work we would be attempting from "Day One".

At Washington University, in St. Louis, where I attended Dental School, I think we were given an outstanding clinical introduction that gave all of us a comfortable degree of confidence as we entered residencies and practices right out of school. The extent of our "non-clinical" training, however, was a single one-semester course taught by a clinical psychologist entitled "Patients Are People, Too." Certainly this is everything that we needed to know about the management of a practice...or maybe it was, in another era. Dental meetings are full of lore on how easy it was to generate success in the "golden years" of Dentistry, when all that was needed was to hang a shingle, "drill, fill and bill". It certainly is not like that now.

Today, dentists everywhere relate struggles and challenges in generating a sufficient amount of treatment to make the practice of dentistry profitable. There are concerns about the economy, practice management, staff management, overhead, schedule management, insurance dependence, government regulations, corporate intervention and financial planning for eventual retirement.

So...what qualifies me as an "expert" to offer the solutions to these challenges? Very little except first, I am a Dentist. I have a BA in Business and Finance from Columbia University. More importantly, I have had an insatiable appetite for Practice Management information from the moment I graduated from Dental School in 1982. While I was a Resident at North Shore University Hospital in Manhasset, NY, and in my early years of practice I went to see every Practice Management "Guru" that I could find. I took notes at every lecture. I listened to every audiocassette and subscribed to and read every newsletter and journal I could put my hands on. With this information, it was pretty easy to create a thriving and profitable practice by the mid 1990's...until the walls started to collapse around me. Then I virtually lost everything.

In 1997 I had a thriving solo practice, approaching $1 million in production. It was starting to become too much for me to manage clinically and otherwise so I incorporated a nearby colleague into my practice as a partner. He was a good dentist with a good reputation, but his practice had stagnated. I mistakenly thought it was a good fit. His hands could help my overload and my practice structure would help him become more productive. I still believe this would have worked had he not withheld the information that he was several years behind on his income taxes. The pressure from collection efforts affected him greatly. His patient care deteriorated and many patients stopped scheduling. His production-based income dropped significantly and he could no longer afford the "buy-in" into our partnership, nor his share of the payments on a $750,000 joint business loan we had taken to renovate and upgrade our facility and practice when we joined into partnership.

In May of 1999 I was sitting at the dinner table in my home on a Thursday evening when the fax line rang. The message was from the fax machine in my office and it indicated that my "partner" was vacating "our" practice so that he could attend to his personal challenges. I immediately raced to my office, only to find that many of my charts were gone, equipment was missing and my computer was pirated. "Our" bank account had been emptied. Two days later I was in an accident and sustained a serious injury that would necessitate multiple surgeries and put me out of work for the better part of the next two years.

I hired dental residents from the hospital where I taught, to "moonlight" in my practice and try to care for my patients on a limited basis. But with less than adequate equipment, few patient charts, a lost computer schedule and no prospect of my returning to work anytime soon, my practice rapidly deteriorated from $1.2 million (in the partnership) to under $300,000. Legal efforts to recoup what was legally owed to me and what had been stolen from me had to be abandoned when the ex-partner declared bankruptcy. This left me with a lost practice, $10,000 per month payments on my now, inherited joint loan, and little chance of doing anything about it until the summer of 2001, when I could, hopefully, return to work. Near the end of August, 2001 I was finally able to return to work on a limited basis. Great news until two weeks later 9/11 entered all of our lives. There was personal loss of life among members of my team. We lost a significant segment from what remained in our practice and our office was essentially shut down for a couple of months.

In 2002 we began to show some recovery until a member of my team was struck by an out-of-control taxicab in Manhattan, while crossing the street. Unfortunately, the young lady lost one leg completely, the partial use of both arms and was in a coma for several months. As troubled as we were in our situation, we felt compelled to do whatever we could to help our team member to rebuild her life. Over the next 6 months my associate and I drew only what we needed to live. Our team members frequently forewent their pay and, with the receipts from our dentistry, we were able to make a significant difference in her life. When she emerged from her coma we were able to pay $135,000 for a computerized prosthetic limb. We handed her $500,000 in cash to help with her astronomic expenses (The driver who had struck her had no insurance and her own medical insurance would not pay since it was the result of an accident.) Then it struck me. Or rather, my family, my associate and what was left of my team confronted me about restoring "our" lives.

I had always been a student of practice management. I absorbed all that I learned. It became time to apply all of those lessons. I developed a vision of the practice I wanted to create. I surrounded myself with an incredible team, of individuals who believed and shared my vision. We acquired training in dental skills, interpersonal skills, verbal skills and emotional well-being. We adopted a structured plan for growth. We implemented and documented clear, defined systems. We learned to trust one another, encourage one another and we incentivized our practice to insure that everyone received financial and emotional fulfillment.

The result is that in a period of 6 years we grew our practice from $300,000 production to over $2.5 million. More importantly, we created a practice with a culture of positivity and fulfillment, fueled by the tremendous amount of cosmetic, implant and life enhancing care that we provide for a practice bursting at the seams with appreciative patients.

This is the story of a practice recovering by overcoming challenges. As I visit practices throughout the New York metropolitan area, I regularly see practices trying to "recover" from challenges incurred during the last few years. My hope is that the stories and ideas offered in this book will help to stimulate, motivate and engage the doctors and team members who read it into adopting some of these ideas into their practices. I hope that these ideas will have a similar positive influence on your practices and that you will also be able to achieve your full potential and become fulfilled emotionally and financially in your practices.

The book is divided into the four main factors, aside from clinical ability, which contribute to the growth and success of a practice. These factors are Leadership, Business Prowess, People Skills and Sales Strategies. While some may insist that Leadership and People Skills are the product of certain personality types, I will counter with the fact that they are traits encompassing learned skills that can be mastered through a constant awareness and conscious application, similar to Business Prowess and Sales Strategies. It is important to understand that these four factors are interrelated on many planes and that there is redundancy, at times, between them. I have not let that deter me from reiterating those themes that I view as particularly important when they have come up in varying contexts.

None of what I discuss is etched in stone as being absolute in either principal or execution. Because of that I welcome feedback at any point along the way as you read through this book. I am very passionate about this material and I love to discuss it, at length. If you have any questions, or comments, please contact me:

Email: smilepotential@aol.com
Cell phone: 516-524-7573

SECTION ONE

What They Taught Us In Dental School About How To Manage A Dental Practice

This page intentionally left blank

This page intentionally left blank

This page intentionally left blank

This page intentionally left blank

SECTION TWO

They Didn't Teach Us That In Dental School

For practical purposes, it has become evident to me through the years that the responsibilities for managing a thriving dental practice fall under four main categories, Leadership, Business Prowess, People, and Sales. Of course, all of these categories overlap on many different planes. Section Two is divided into these four categories to enable there to be a feeling of concentration and consistency as each of them are described. The categorization is loose and within each category there will be some redundancy. Hopefully, repetition will give credibility to some of the ideas as being relatively more important than some of the others. Constantly give importance to some of the key words, Vision, Value and Appreciation.

Category One: Leadership

CHAPTER 1

Taking Control In a World
That is Out of Our Control

The headlines during the course of the last few years have certainly emphasized the point that the world around us is out of our control. We have endured terrible storms with unprecedented flooding, tree damage, loss of homes and property, and prolonged power outages. We have seen senseless carnage from deranged misfits in Newtown and Aurora. We have been frustrated by the inability of our elected officials to practice compromise to enact meaningful change for everyone. We are bombarded with news stories of problems with our economy and in world politics. This all makes it very clear that we are virtually helpless in controlling our surroundings. We can vote one way or another, reinforce our physical environment and insure ourselves "up the wazoo", and we can go about our life with constant caution, but the fact of the matter is, "You never know".

In our practices, however, we have the ability to take control. While we need to be cognizant of the world around us, too often we are paralyzed by concern for circumstances over which we have no control and which do not directly affect us on a daily basis. As long as a situation does not directly affect us, we need to focus all of our energy and effort on the factors over which we do have control. We absolutely do control our level of success and fulfillment. Hope is not a strategy. When times become challenging we should not "wait for the storm to pass" but, rather, we should "learn to dance in the rain". During the past four years I have spoken to too many dentists who are frustrated by the course of events and are "riding it out" until conditions improve. This strategy will always fail. Easy success and prosperity prior to 2008 bred complacency in our levels of efficiency and leadership. The economy did not cause the problems in our practices. It has just magnified the problems that were there. The things that we could get by with when the economy was good, we can't get by with now.

We need to critically evaluate every single thing that we do within our practices. More importantly, we need to accept the challenge to become leaders in our practices. Not clinical leaders or financial leaders. We need to become cultural and emotional leaders in order to maintain the enthusiasm and motivation of the members of our teams. Nearly every dentist I have met has had the clinical skills to become successful. Unfortunately clinical skill does not ultimately determine the level of success that most dentists achieve. I have seen far too many with Pankey, Dawson and LVI training struggling to maintain the viability of their practices because of inadequate leadership skills.

One of the true statesmen of our time is Mr. Robert Gates, who was a University President, Director of the CIA and the Secretary of Defense under Presidents Bush and Obama. At a recent leadership conference Mr. Gates was asked, "What does it take to be a leader?" Without any hesitation, Mr. Gates responded, "Take care of the people under you."

In our practices we need to "take care" of our team members. Respect their commitments to family and faith. That is the reason they work, just as it should be for the doctors. Expect them to perform to the highest level that they have been trained. Training is key to their performance. Inadequate training and unrealistic expectations based on their level of training is the main reason for inadequate performance. Invest time and increased resources on the training of your teams. Recognize and acknowledge their performance at EVERY opportunity. This seems to be a tremendous challenge for so many doctors that I have met with. Acknowledgement is the most important need of our team members as long as they are adequately compensated. Learn how to offer constructive criticism, when necessary, in a way that builds the self-esteem of your team members instead of destroying it. When you set an example in this area, you will empower your team to act the same way with their coworkers. This will prevent gossiping and facilitate accountability to each other in finding solutions instead of problems. Learn to respond to setbacks instead of reacting. This applies to situations in our personal lives as well as in our practices.

The years ahead will be as challenging as the past few. We have no control over the world and the economy around us. With this being said, we do have control over our ultimate levels of professional success. Learn the tenets of leadership and you will feel less "out of control".

CHAPTER 2

Strive for Perfection, Accept Excellence

When I speak to audiences I am generally faced with two types of doctors and team members. There are those who defensively assert that they do everything that I talk about and there are others who appreciate reminders of things that they do and welcome additional ideas for improvement. Those who insist that they do everything; I usually find that they do very little; though they may have done some variation at a time in the past. They dismiss the information and leave with no intention of changing anything. They keep doing the same things and, consequently, they keep getting the same results.

Those on the other side of the aisle in my presentations often sit there nodding their heads in affirmation and feel proud that they have made an effort to try new things and welcome even the smallest pearls for improvement. They welcome change and accept the fact that nothing is wasted if something new does not work. I recently attended a forum where former President Bill Clinton spoke. His advice to the young people in the audience was that, "It is better to try and fail than to never have tried." Some of the great minds of the past century failed in early attempts to be innovative. Colonel Sanders took his recipe for fried chicken to 100 restaurants before he opened up his own restaurant, which later became KFC. Steven Jobs was fired by Apple years before he rejoined the company and inspired Apple's unprecedented success. Fred Smith was told his MBA thesis at the Warton Business School, which described a hub-based delivery system to insure overnight delivery anywhere in the country, was ridiculous and he received a failing grade. Then he left the University of Pennsylvania and founded Federal Express. Thomas Edison, one of the greatest inventors in US history once said, "I have not failed 10,000 times. I have not failed once. I have merely succeeded in proving that those 10,000 ways will not work. When I have eliminated the ways that will not work, I will find the way that will."

I encourage change in the practices that I work with. Constant change is necessary in the pursuit of excellence. But is it enough? At my 30th Dental School reunion in St Louis, Dr. Brick Sheer, a classmate of mine from Kansas City, Missouri, told me that the motto for he and his team is "We strive for perfection, but accept excellence." Do you think Brick is constantly trying out new strategies and systems? You betcha! There is no greater virtue than the pursuit of excellence.

In the words of the famous football coach, Vince Lombardi, "The quality of a man's life is in direct proportion to his commitment to excellence, regardless of his chosen field of endeavor." As you strive for perfection in your practices, you will reap the benefits of welcoming excellence.

CHAPTER 3

Mirror, Mirror On the Wall...

I t is a very good strategy to retrospectively review the year just passed in the world around us, in our profession, in our offices and in our lives. It's always timely to evaluate what was satisfying, what was disappointing, what changed and what we'd like to change.

The world around us is in turmoil. There is widespread political and economic unrest. Those in positions to make change seem unable to agree on solutions. Thus, little seems to get accomplished. While we must be aware of what is occurring around us, we must realize that most of it is out of our control and not exhaust needless energies on these problems.

Our profession is undergoing rapid change. There has been a widespread acceptance of digital technology in our treatment rooms. There has been a sudden explosion in the use of social media as a marketing tool and educational forum. There has been a drastic change in patient behavior, which has necessitated a change in how we do business in order to be successful. And there are questions about how the case of the FTC suing the North Carolina State Board of Dental Examiners will transform dentistry from a profession into

a trade, not just for bleaching, but also for other procedures in the future. This, too, is out of our control.

In our practices it is a time to evaluate how we did in
the previous 12 months. Did we exceed or fail to meet
expectations? Did we even have expectations? How
has it been? We have been in many practices where
recent times have been very challenging. We have also
been in practices where the previous 12 months was
their best year ever. More importantly, it is necessary to
evaluate what contributed to successes or failures. I do
not mean throwing your hands up and saying "it was the
economy." It is critical to be more analytical and use
practice statistics to determine, based on what hap-
pened, what each of us could have done to have made
a difference and change the ultimate result. It's important to create an awareness that you have to work on
your practice as well as in it.

One of the tools we may use is to hold performance
reviews for the members of our teams. A performance
review is not related to a compensation review. A performance review is a tool to evaluate what a team member is doing well, what is expected of them, what they
can improve upon and a discussion of what is preventing them from achieving at a higher level with an eye on
the next 12 months as a period for positive change and
development.

Just as it is important to evaluate the performance of
the members of our team, it is imperative to evaluate the
performance of the doctor. Self-evaluation in addition to

evaluations from key team members can be a difficult nut to swallow for some doctors. However, more than any other individual, the performance of the doctor can make or break a practice. Has the doctor exhibited strong leadership? In my seminars I speak about the "Leader's Challenge". The "Leaders Challenge" is to create a clear vision for the practice with defined expectations and goals for every aspect of your practice. Then, the intent is to inspire and motivate the team to come on board and enjoy the ride. Third, is to lead by example. If we expect our team members to make changes, we must be equally willing to do the same, or we risk sabotaging our own practices. And lastly, we must be willing to encourage our team members and show appreciation for jobs well done.

Are you, the doctors, equipped to take the pulse of your practices, to determine who does what well, measure performance and reassign responsibilities, based on strengths and weaknesses? Is your office computerized and are you using your management system to the full extent that it is capable of? Are there 2 or 3 new services that your practice can offer? Are there technologies with an immediate return on investment that you can incorporate which provide a great service and generate revenue, such as Velscope? Are you committed to learning about marketing and promotion of your practice? Have you become internet-savvy? Are you fostering open and constructive communication among your team with daily huddles and weekly meetings?

Have you eliminated the blinders that can limit treatment to one tooth at a time and, instead, adopted a belief system based on more thorough patient evaluation and more comprehensive treatment presentation? Are you strategically managing overhead to secure a profit that will assure you financial security when you will no longer be practicing? Are you taking time to do things for yourself to insure health, wellness and happiness with those who mean the most to you?

There is so much to consider and so much you can change for the better if you look in the mirror.

"I'm starting with the Man in the Mirror.
I'm asking him to change his ways.
And no message could have been any clearer.
If you wanna make the world (or practice, or life)
a better place,
If you wanna make the world (or practice, or life)
a better place,
Take a look at yourself, and then make a
change.
Take a look at yourself, and then make a
change.
Na Na Na, Na Na Na, Na Na, Na Na"

—Michael Jackson, 1988.

If this challenge seems daunting, seek the help of a mentor or Coach. Change can be difficult without the help of others.

CHAPTER 4

Play Ball and Evaluate Your Roster!

As a lifelong baseball fan and a loyal fan of the New York Mets since their first season at the Polo Grounds, recent seasons have been very disappointing. Their general lack of experience, lack of fundamentals and a confused, distracted ownership remind me of some of the challenges that I have seen in some dental practices in recent months.

One of the first questions I frequently ask dentists is "Which comes first, quality dentistry or prosperity?" Most of the dentists I visit insist that they practice quality dentistry and are confused why this does not automatically lead to prosperity. Unfortunately, we have seen firsthand that some of the best-trained and most talented dentists are not necessarily the most highly compensated.

The challenge is to create a vision for the practice that emphasizes an elevation in the perceived value to the patients of every aspect of the services provided in the practice. The first steps in this process are creation of the vision, communicating the vision to the team and developing a degree of professionalism in the members of the team, second to none. It is imperative to fight the pressures of commoditization and to look at how we can evolve the quality of the service we provide so that the practice can begin to attract and develop patients who are interested in cosmetic and comprehensive care and who see the value of creating independence from the constraints of their insurance benefits.

In looking for examples of the degree of professionalism that we need it is painful for this Mets fan to look in the Bronx for the finest example of professionalism in baseball, Derek Jeter, who recently announced his retirement.

Derek Jeter possesses a vision of excellence; a strong work ethic and leadership that seems to constantly make the other members of his team perform better. If we are to exercise a vision of excellence we must resist the temptations to use cheap dental labs that farm their work to foreign dental mills with no quality control. We must resist the temptation to hire the lowest paid team members and exercise patience to hire articulate, refined individuals who show a desire to want to constantly learn and improve their ability to reflect the pursuit of excellence. Carefully observe how Derek Jeter not only performs well on the field, but he also sets a good example off the field. He carefully calculates his words and commentary to constantly paint his teammates and organization in the best possible light, without ever making excuses or placing blame on others for unsatisfactory results. Develop scripts for your team members so that they are promoting and raising the perceived value of your care in every opportunity that they have in speaking with patients and prospective patients.

Another attribute of Derek Jeter is the way that he exudes "Yankee Pride". He values the symbolism of his pinstripes the way that I would like to see dental team members valuing the vision and belief systems of their practices. When I survey dental team members as to the qualities they appreciate in their practices, too often I hear that "it's close to my home" or "the hours are convenient". Even worse is when I see dentists saying the same things. I suggest polling your team members and find out what it is that they value in their employment in your practices. Those that mention simple convenience or social reasons are not the team members that you can depend on to fuel the future growth and development of your practice. Identify the team members that share your vision of helping people, making a difference in people's lives and participating in the delivery of the highest quality care possible. Grant incentives to those team members, who constantly look to improve their performance, take on additional responsibility and increase the practice's profitability and surround them with other team members who will share in these initiatives. If you are able to develop all-stars at every position, players like Derek Jeter, then your victories will mount and in time you will develop your own dental dynasty.

CHAPTER 5

Who Wants to Be A Millionaire?

O n the popular game show, *Who Wants To Be A Millionaire*, contestants are granted three lifelines to help them with the answers to questions where they lack certainty. The first lifeline is limiting the possible choices to two, thus giving a 50% chance of answering the question correctly. The second lifeline is phoning a friend; hopefully an expert on the topic of the question, and the third lifeline is asking the audience for their consensus. The ultimate goal is to answer enough questions correctly to earn $1,000,000. It seems very similar to the quest that many dentists have in their practices.

In our practices, we, too, are granted lifelines in our quest to earn our dream. Our teams, if they have been empowered, serve as the first lifeline. They facilitate limiting our options by helping us to formulate a practice vision. We place a huge importance on the creation of a clear vision, not as an exercise, but, more importantly, as a template for all of the decisions that we make in the daily operation of a practice. Do we choose to take insurance, or not? Do we choose to emphasize quality, service or affordability? Do we choose to invest in technology? In theory, these possible choices are limited by the vision we have created for our practice **with** our team members.

The most popular lifeline that the majority of us depend on is "phoning a friend". By surrounding ourselves with great advisors, hopefully we have amassed experts in every aspect of our practice. Whether we depend on mentors, colleagues, accountants, attorneys, computer experts or our dental sales reps, we have numerous individuals with a wealth of knowledge in our field to help us make the best decisions for our practices.

I believe that the most valuable lifeline is our audience, or in the case of our dental practices, the patients we serve. Through the years our practice, Smiles On Broadway, has assembled a series of **Patient Advisory Councils** (PACs). A Patient Advisory Council is essentially a focus group of patients who are willing to give us honest feedback on their perceptions of our practice, whether it is positive or negative. Some may think that surveys serve as an adequate method of gaining feedback. I argue that it is the interaction of the patients with our team and with each other that gives this concept its credibility.

Which patients do we ask to participate? Our team nominates patients who they think will be willing to give us feedback...period. Some of them may be our "best patients", but of greater value are patients who may offer suggestions, or even criticism. We have even invited patients who have left our practice for one reason or another. We generously reward the patients who come so even past patients find it worthwhile to attend.

We choose a fine dining restaurant whose service mirrors the exemplary service we feel we offer in our practice. We have hosted as many as 20 and as few as 12 patients. After wine and hors d'eouvres we sit at a large table where everyone can see everyone else. We include 2 or 3 team members in the meeting to sit (separated) among the patients. After the first course and a brief introduction the patients are asked, in turn, to comment on things they like or appreciate about our practice. Many will speak about a wonderful experience or result that they have had. This is the portion of the meeting that feels good. Even the past patients relay some positive thoughts.

After the main course, we ask attendees to comment on something about our practice that disappointed them or something they would like to see different. This is the most important part of the meeting. God gave us two ears and one mouth and this is the part of the meeting to use them in just that ratio. Listen and validate every comment, no matter how trivial or off base they may seem. These are the people you serve and their perceptions will ultimately make or break your practice. As you listen to them and validate them they begin to become empowered as missionaries for the practice. They become personally involved in the desire to make your practice successful. The attendees, who we refer to as our "Board of Directors", begin to become our very best source of referrals and those who had previously left the practice, often return. After the fact, be sure to keep attendees informed about your progress in implementing their suggestions and solutions to their complaints. The follow through to their input is what raises their loyalty to an unprecedented level. As Jeffrey Gitomer said in his book of the same title, "Patient satisfaction is worthless. Patient loyalty is priceless." The creation of this level of patient loyalty may be just what is necessary to help you become a millionaire...if that's what you want.

CHAPTER 6

Hope Is Not A Strategy

When I question dentists mid-year about what is going on in their practices, many describe abbreviated schedules, weekends off and vacations. Nothing could make me happier. It is important to recharge our batteries and I faithfully subscribe to the notion that we "work to live and not live to work". But, in a similar vein, we have heard dentists describe open time in their schedules, fewer new patients and declining production. When we ask what is being done about these circumstances, the response we get is that it's the summer and "we'll refocus after Labor Day".

This procrastination can be damaging to a practice. July marks the end of the first half of the year. It should be a time to analyze the trends within the practice, which metrics are improving, and which ones are not. It is a time to begin planning for the strategies that we will implement after Labor Day. If we wait until Labor Day to begin mobilizing it will create a significant lag in what we can do and it may prevent meaningful changes from taking place. "If you fail to plan, then you plan to fail."

Use the summer to review the Vision for the practice. Review what has worked and what has not. Add to and tweak the practices and strategies that have worked and change the ones which have not. Develop your marketing plan for the last third of the year, including the establishment of a promotional budget. Develop strategies to promote some of the elective procedures you enjoy doing and which add to the revenue of your practice. Planning a systematic approach along with the development of beliefs and purpose will make your practices magnets for success.

CHAPTER 7

Make This Year Your Super Bowl Year

Having worked with the New York Jets for quite a few seasons, Super Bowl XLVI in 2012 was a difficult one to watch...until it dawned on me that the New York Giants season could be a model for all of us in our dental practices.

First of all, the preparation for their season was inadequate due to the lockout-shortened pre-season. In our practices, there is often inadequate preparation for success. We should all be sitting down with our teams in the beginning of the year and planning our course, setting goals, conducting performance reviews and refining our vision for the year.

There were injuries to numerous key Giants players that prevented some from suiting up and others from performing at a peak level. The disappointing early performance created a negative culture of doubt in the clubhouse. Some of our team members also suffer injuries, though not physical in nature. Excessive criticism and a lack of positive feedback can create a lack of confidence and a reluctance to take initiative to independently function at a high level. Our practices may have a negative culture that is felt by the patients as well as by you and the rest of the team. First of all, ELIMINATE GOSSIP and pay attention to conditions which may adversely affect the emotional atmosphere in your practice. Devote time every day to give positive feedback and acknowledge each and every member of your team for his or her efforts on your behalf.

For the Giants, there was much doubt about the lack of leadership exhibited by Coach Coughlin and many were calling for his dismissal. Fortunately for many in our profession, the owner and the leader are one in the same and it's unlikely the dentist would fire himself. But just as we spend time on developing our clinical skills, it is equally important for us to develop our leadership skills. In addition to showing appreciation to our team members we must clearly define the vision for our team, lead by example and motivate and inspire everyone to help pedal our practices in the same direction.

The Giants heard constant discouragement from the media and their fans. There were boos from fans during a 4-game losing streak. The external factors created a need to dig down deep and overcome the doom and gloom naysayers. The dental profession is also facing some external pressures. We have insurance companies constantly trying to force our reimbursements down and trying to make many feel that insurance subservience is necessary to succeed. The media is a constant source of discouragement as we hear the troubling news about the economy, unemployment, taxes and the recession. We need to stop focusing on the elements that we cannot control and focus 100% of our effort on the elements that we can control, our leadership, our team's development, our vision, our verbal skills and our clinical skills.

Finally, we must applaud the resilience, the effort, the skill and the qualities that made the Giants successful in winning the Lombardi Trophy in Super Bowl XLVI. They did not listen to the negative predictions. They had a clearly defined vision and goals. They developed a solid "game plan". They practiced hard. They believed in each other. They executed well. And they had the good fortune to have some luck on their side.

This is exactly what we need to do in our practices. Remain aware of what is occurring that may affect our practices but be equally aware that there are practices that are achieving tremendous success, nevertheless. Focus on the systems and strategies that you have defined that will bring success to your practice. Develop clarity in your vision and allow the vision to help you make day-to-day decisions that will bring you closer to that goal. Focus on the development of your team and begin each day with a huddle to make sure every member of your team "knows the proper routes" to run throughout the day. Practice your systems regularly with ongoing training and roleplaying to master the verbal skills necessary to achieve success in raising the perceived value of care in your practice. Develop a belief in each member of your team and focus on creating a positive, encouraging, and mutually rewarding culture. Have fun! And if you can do all of these things, with a little luck, you too will be on your way to YOUR Super Bowl and you and your team, and your patients will be World Champions.

Category Two: Business

CHAPTER 8

Defining Success

The mission that I established for Smile Potential five years ago was to help dentists and their teams realize the full potential of their practices and enjoy the success of realizing that potential. What does that mean?

An American business consultant was standing on the pier of a small Mexican fishing village during a much-needed vacation. It was his first vacation in over 10 years because of the demands of his job. He noticed that a small boat with just one fisherman was pulling up to the dock and inside his boat were several large fin tunas. The consultant complimented the fisherman on his catch and asked him how long it had taken to catch them.

The Mexican replied, *"Only a little while."*

The consultant then asked, *"Why didn't you stay out longer and catch more fish?"*

The Mexican replied, *"I have enough to support my family for a little while."*

The consultant then asked, *"What do you do with the rest of your time?"*

The Mexican fisherman said, *"I sleep late, fish a little, play with my children, take siestas with my wife, and stroll into the village each evening where I sip wine and play my guitar with my amigos. I have a full and busy life."*

The consultant scoffed, *"I have a Harvard MBA and I can help you. You should spend more time fishing and with the proceeds, buy a bigger boat and with the proceeds from the bigger boat you could buy several boats. Eventually you would have a fleet of fishing boats. Instead of selling your catch to a middleman you would sell it to a processor and eventually open your own cannery. You would be able to control the product, the processing and the distribution. You would leave this small coastal fishing village and move to Mexico City and eventually, New York, where you would run the expanding business from the corner office in a high-rise office building."*

The Mexican fisherman asked, *"How long will all of this take?"* The American replied, *"Approximately 15-20 years."* The Mexican asked, *"But what then?"*

The American laughed and said that's the best part. *"When the time is right you will announce an IPO and sell your company stock to the public and become very rich. You will make millions of dollars."*

The Mexican then asked, *"Millions of dollars? Then what?"*

The American said, *"Then you would retire and move to a small coastal fishing village where you would sleep late, fish a little, play with your grandkids, take siestas with your wife, and stroll into the village each evening where you could sip wine and play your guitar with your amigos."*

There are many ways to define success. Becoming a successful dentist depends on YOUR definition of success. For some it is having a practice with many patients and making lots of money. Having two or more offices and several associates is a mark of success for others. Some dentists may prefer to have a smaller practice where they get to know each patient personally and treat all members of the same family. Others, still, may feel that a successful practice alleviates the fear that many people have of dentistry or that it brings change to peoples' conditions and makes a difference in their lives. One problem is that many think their success is tied to an unfounded belief that their worth is based solely on how successful their dental practice is and that they cannot control that with any certainty.

Success occurs by design, not by accident. It is natural to look for ways to make our practices and our lives better. It is important to be deliberate in taking actions to strive for improvement. Hope is not a strategy. It is important to make a commitment to identify strategies that bring about positive change and then to practice a high degree of consistency to repeat those strategies. When you can identify these actions and activities, and can repeat them on a regular basis, whether it be with clinical skills, relationships and communication, goals and a vision in harmony with your core values, professionalism exhibited by you and your team, cleanliness of your facility, office procedures and protocols, marketing and advertising, equipment and technology, or management methods and style, you hold the power over the momentum you develop towards achieving success and happiness.

There are many components to the success we achieve in dentistry. Clinical success is established by providing a high level of care that provides years of problem-free service. Financial success is the easiest to quantify. If you want a "million dollar practice" it's easy to calculate what daily and monthly production will get you there. Respect of peers and community is a measure of success that is hard to measure, but it is enhanced by a willingness to help others learn what you know. Loyalty and respect from patients is something we never measure and many dentists often take it for granted. It is totally reactionary. We know how it feels when a long-time patient requests that their records be sent to another practice. We also know how good it feels when a patient thanks us for our effort or recommends us to a friend. Pride of accomplishment is an indicator of success when we finish a challenging case and know that it looks great, feels comfortable and will serve the patient for many years. Finally, there is the personal fulfillment of all of the above and many other aspects of spending wonderful days enjoying the use current technology with a great team in caring for appreciative patients. Dentistry is a wonderful profession with many rewards. Unfortunately, many dentists spend their careers, and their lives, disappointed, unhappy and unfulfilled. It does not have to be that way. Define YOUR success, both professionally and personally, and commit to achieving your potential.

CHAPTER 9

SOOT-SOT-GOOT

The beginning of each year is a time when we resolve to change something that will result in a positive effect on our lives. It should also be the time to resolve to make a similar type of change in our practices. I would suggest that each practice's first resolution for any year should be **SOOT - SOT - GOOT.**

There is not a single strategy that can have more of an impact on a practice. It is the number one marketing strategy. If it is not done, it can be the number one disappointment to our patients. It is the number one turnoff from a previous practice that patients describe when they join a new practice. Remember that every new patient was the patient of another dentist before they came to your office. It affects patient satisfaction, employee harmony and office culture unlike anything else that we do, or fail to do.

SOOT – SOT – GOOT is:
1) **S**tart **O**ut **O**n **T**ime!
2) **S**tay **O**n **T**ime!
3) **G**et **O**ut **O**n **T**ime!

To not practice **SOOT - SOT - GOOT** reflects a breakdown in a system or, worse, a lack of a system. It shows a disregard and disrespect for patients' time and team members' schedules. It has a negative effect on ultimate production and discourages referrals of new patients.

So how do we accomplish **SOOT - SOT - GOOT**? Here is a partial *Action Plan* to help make it happen:

- Establish a policy that tardiness will not be tolerated from any member of the team, doctor included. There should be consequences for lateness. For team members, it might be forfeiture of any daily bonus for the day, or even dismissal, if it persists for an extended time. Remember the uncooperative late team member puts an added burden on other members of the team and breeds resentment. For the doctor, it could be the team not turning on the lights or not preparing treatment rooms for the first patient until the doctor has participated in the morning huddle.
- Practice efficient time management by doing procedure time studies for each common procedure performed by the doctor and hygienist. Take each procedure that you do (i.e.: Molar root canal, single unit crown, MOD posterior resin) and time that procedure from start to finish four to six times and then calculate the average time needed to complete the procedure. Take into account the difference in time needed for upper

or lower teeth and factor that into your procedure times.

- Keep schmoozing to a minimum or add extra time to procedures to allow for it.
- Do not extend appointments to do extra treatment unless your administrative team concurs. They are the ones that have to deal with patients waiting extended periods of time after showing up on time for appointments.
- Emergency or unforeseen complications are excused under this policy, but the doctor should go out to the waiting patient to apologize and explain the situation. The patient should be given an opportunity to reschedule and some consideration should be given to them for their inconvenience. We recommend a small courtesy for their rescheduled appointment or a simple $5 Dunkin Donuts or Starbucks gift card is a nice touch.
- At the end of the day DO NOT go beyond your scheduled hours. Patients do not really appreciate being treated longer than for the time they had expected. They associate unplanned longer appointments with things not going as planned and it affects their confidence. Patients have outside plans and family commitments and they resent missing these occasions. More important, it is a tremendous imposition on team members. They certainly have lives outside the office and that should be the priority in their lives, whether

the doctor agrees or not. Respect their time and their commitments and they will support you when you truly need them. If a true emergency requires that treatment extend beyond the scheduled hours, please be sure to first ask the team member, not expect them to stay, and then pay them time-and-a-half for a significantly extended appointment or some other reward for helping you to become more profitable.

- Finally, conduct a team meeting to discuss this strategy. The operative word is "discuss". Discuss what the practice experience has been. Discuss all of the things that would have to change in order to make **SOOT – SOT – GOOT** happen and then how each member of the team would feel about the changes. Team members want to be heard and want to feel that they have been a part of change. Validate them and they will begin to help drive the practice to new heights. The meeting should be scheduled and the team should be made aware of what will be discussed ahead of time. And just as everything else, with this meeting, START OUT ON TIME, STAY ON TIME AND GET OUT ON TIME!

CHAPTER 10

Who's Counting?

As I travel around visiting offices, one of the first questions I ask dentists is to tell me how their practices are doing. Inevitably the answers tend to be conceptual; good, not so good, terrible. Rarely do dentists know more than a vague interpretation of how they "think" their practices are performing. When I try to be more specific in my questioning, such as asking about even the most basic measurable statistics, such as Production, Collection, A/R, New Patients, so many dentists are completely in the dark. This lack of awareness prevents dentists from developing strategies to grow their practices and overcome economic trends. In different eras, when success could be achieved in the absence of strategy and systems, complacency could be explained by the cliché, "If knowledge is power, then ignorance is bliss." Currently, few dentists who are practicing blindly are experiencing much bliss.

Unconditionally, Dentists, Office Managers and all members of the dental team must maintain an ongoing awareness and understanding of the measurable events in their practices. These functions include Production, Collection, Accounts Receivable, New Patients,

Overhead Percent, Break-even point and Production per hour.

In looking at Production and Collection, trends are as important as the monthly figures. The chart below shows the two-year production for a typical dental practice. The straight line indicates the general trend of production.

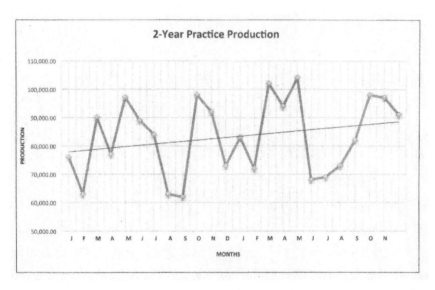

Whenever we plot the production of a practice, inevitably we are going to see peaks and valleys. We find it easy to explain the valleys; vacations, illness, inclement weather, catastrophic events. The peaks should be viewed as the potential of the practice. The question we must ask when looking at a chart like this is "what prevented the practice from sustaining the peaks?" If a practice is capable of achieving these levels, then if we can duplicate this achievement in successive months, ultimately the trend-line will begin to reflect a period of sustained growth. Often times we find

that achieving these months of high production intro-
duces new and different types of stress to the practice.
This stress can usually be attributed to a lack of systems
or the inadequacy of systems, if there are systems in
place. With this information, strategic planning should
be directed to revising or tweaking systems that will
allow for increased production in subsequent periods.

I find that the best statistic in measuring the efficiency of a practice is the hourly production of each
provider. It is an easy measurement to compute and
should be readjusted each month. A good way of calcu-
lating production per hour is to calculate the total production and hours worked for each provider for each of
the last three months and then employ a weighted average to make the number more relevant at that particular
point in time. Hygienists will typically average between
$100 and $250 per hour. We have seen Doctors in difficult situations averaging as low as $200 per hour. Most
of the Doctors we work with have elevated to the $600-
900 level and we have seen some Doctors increase to
producing as much as $1,200-1,500 per hour.

The advantage of directing your practice through the
understanding of production per hour is that small
adjustments, when compounded, can have a major
impact on production over a period of time.

On the next page I have given 4 examples of how
modest goals for increased production can impact on
the hourly production and significantly increase your
bottom line.

DOCTOR	HYGIENIST
1 Additional resin/day ($200) Results in $25/hour increase Yearly increase is $40,000	1 Additional sealant/day ($40) Results in $5/hour increase Yearly increase is $8,000
1 additional crown/day ($1,000) Results in $125/hour increase Yearly increase is $200,000	1 additional Root Plane/day ($160) Results in $20/hour increase Yearly increase is $300,000

Accomplishing these increases must be a total team effort. The new patient and all existing patients must be indoctrinated into the concept of comprehensive diagnosis. The focus of promoting this level of more comprehensive care becomes the result of enhancing the patient experience, raising their perceived value of the care they are receiving and explaining all treatment, not in terms of the treatment being rendered, but more importantly, in the context of the benefit of the care to the patient.

The process of elevating your practice to new levels of achievement, once again, begins with raising your awareness of the basic measurable events within your practice. Then, the interpretation of these metrics helps to guide the practice and the entire team to strategically plan changes by setting modest reachable new goals for production, which when compounded over the course of the year will have a major impact in helping the practice reach and maintain new levels of achievement.

CHAPTER 11

Realize The Full Potential Of Your Computer

I recently attended the User's Conference for my office's Management and Charting Software System with three members from my team. I have sincere regrets that I have never attended this meeting before. My office has been computerized since 1985. We have had the present system since 1997. While we utilize a great deal of what our system has to offer, much of what we do is based on how we set it up originally in 1997. For 17 years I have been blessed with a dedicated, inspired and motivated team, who have constantly strived for better or more efficient ways to use our system. Where I have let them down is by not feeding their curiosity by giving them sufficient exposure to the newer developments within our system. It was thrilling to see how excited and inspired they were, and how much they learned, from attending this meeting.

As I visit offices in and around the metropolitan area, I am disappointed with the under-utilization of the office computer systems. I've been in offices where systems have not been used at all since they were installed for various reasons. More commonly, I see offices using systems with wonderful capabilities for only a few basic tasks or duplicating computer functions with concurrent manual systems. Whether it is a failure in proper installation causing tremendous early frustrations, or insufficient training leading to a lack of confidence on the part of the team, or a long-time team member resisting change and even sabotaging computer utilization to maintain a status quo with inefficient, but comfortable manual systems, the lack of computer utilization prevents the practice from becoming more efficient and more profitable.

An office using an Information Technology (IT) person who is experienced in working on computers, but who has never installed Dental Software often causes the first problem. Dental Software is more complex than the software used in almost any other field. If your IT person is not experienced with Dental Software, the chances are you WILL have problems with a server-based system. For this reason, we heartily recommend Scott Sanford and his company, *Healthy IT (healthyit.net)* as a great resource person for the computerization of Dental Practices. Scott works with ONLY dental practices, over a hundred of them, and he is tremendously familiar with all of the major dental software systems. We have personally recommended him to over 40 practices and we receive nothing but praise and thanks for the referral. If you would like to speak with Scott, you may call him at *631-224-9450*, or email him at *sts@stsanford.com*.

How many practices have high-speed handpieces with a capability of hundreds of thousands of revolutions per minute, yet only use low speed handpieces or limit the high speed to 20-40,000 rpm? Well this is exactly what offices are doing by not letting their computers loose and utilizing them to their full potential. Our computer systems have the ability to create a WOW first impression to new patients. They allow us to more accurately and efficiently perform comprehensive patient evaluations. They significantly aid our ability to construct impressive case presentations and increase patient acceptance of comprehensive care. They allow us to schedule more efficiently and more important, productively. They allow us to more efficiently manage the receivables of our practices so that we collect what we produce. And they allow us to dramatically improve the communication with our existing and future patients and create interest and inspiration in their desire for dental care in our practices.

When we attended the User's Conference for our system there were many excellent lectures on how to use new features, or existing features more efficiently. More importantly, there were an unlimited number of support and training representatives available for one-on-one time to trouble-shoot problems and remotely tap into office systems to reconfigure existing modules and increase practice capabilities. The bottom line is that I highly recommend that every office attend the User's Conference for their system when it is scheduled next. Call your software company to find out what is planned. Meet with representative of your systems at regional dental meetings. Experience has shown that attendance at many of the dental meetings has been down in recent years and if this is the case, your rep or one of the support team or trainers will have more time to sit with you and give individualized help and support in helping you realize the full potential of your system.

CHAPTER 12

Overcoming Fee Resistance

Remember that whenever a patient responds to a treatment presentation with a question it is a sign that they are interested in receiving care. It is a call to your action because they just need help in overcoming some challenge. The five most common objections are Cost, Fear, Time, Sense of Urgency and Trust. These objections, therefore, are opportunities to enlist the patient in treatment.

The most common objection is cost. The first strategy in overcoming fee-resistance is to find out if it is the total cost, or if it would be workable if it was fit into a monthly cash flow. If this seems workable, then the patient is a candidate to enroll in third party interest-free financing with a company like CareCredit.

Here are some quotes to incorporate into the discussion:

"It is best to explain a fee once rather than apologize for quality forever."

"We realize people forget price, but never forget poor quality."

"The bitterness of poor quality lasts longer than the sweetness of a low price."

"Our treatment plans are not based on cost or diffi-culty. They are based on the best long-term solution for you."

"The choice we make is to do the best, hire the best and use the best, rather than end up with "get by" results."

CHAPTER 13

Analyze Your Referrals

It is important, in referral relationships, that both offices reflect similar values and standards of care. When a general dentist refers a patient to a dental specialist, the experience in the specialist's office is a reflection on the referring doctor, and vice versa.

I encourage general dentists to sit down with each of the specialists they refer to and discuss what is important to them in the referral relationship. Just as scripting builds patient confidence by unifying the message among members of an office team, coordinating philosophies and treatment explanations between the GP and Specialist also builds confidence and trust. Discuss the importance of communication, treatment coordination and reciprocal referrals. While collegial friendships are great, base referrals on these factors as much as possible. If a patient relates a negative experience at the office of the specialist, call them and discuss it. Don't just sweep it under the rug. If you know how much the patient feels comfortable in your office, channel referrals to specialists whose offices mirror the level of caring, sophistication, policies, and even, the decor of your office. This will raise the perceived value of care that the patient has in the services that you provide to them.

CHAPTER 14

The Best Practice Management Advice Is <u>Free</u>

Many practices have been describing gaps in their schedule, yet the dentists fail to take advantage of a wonderful opportunity to grow their practices. A very astute office manager recently described a scenario that seems to be replicated in many practices. When there is a cancellation or open appointment, the dentist may hide in his or her private office checking emails or net surfing. What happens when a dental sales "rep" enters the reception room? The "rep" identifies himself and asks if the doctor can spend a few moments speaking to him about a new product. The office manager goes into the doctor's office and the dentist says, "Tell them I'm with a patient and I will be with them for a long time." The office manager relays the message to the sales "rep" and they leave some literature and depart the office.

I insist that this practice should be stopped immediately. Dental sales representatives have a wealth of practice management information. They are experts in our field, or at least the good ones are. I do a lot of business with Henry Schein. I like working with Schein because, unlike the discounted mail or web-order suppliers, they have extremely knowledgeable "reps" that visit my office on a regular basis. I have presented programs to the Schein sales team and we have witnessed how they are trained to not "sell" to their clients, but rather listen to the needs of the practice and help to guide them into good business decisions with an eye on maintaining a strong return on investment. The dental sales "reps" visit a minimum of 75-100 offices a month. They see what's working and they see what's not working. They are in an ideal position to give advice to each and every one of us on strategies that we can all use to grow our practices.

We recommend to our clients that they embrace every dental sales "rep" that comes to their office. If the dentist is not with a patient, it should be a no-brainer. If they are with a patient, ask the rep to return during an open time or during a lunch period. When the representative returns, listen to what they have to say about their products and then hire them as a free knowledgeable practice management consultant. When they are completed with their brief pitch, ask to exchange roles and ask them the following question:

"_____(Rep's name), I appreciate you bringing me this information about your products. I am going to think about how I might incorporate them into my practice. In the meantime, I know that you are in quite a few dental practices every week. Could you please tell me 3 things that you have seen other practices doing during the past month that you think might help us to grow or provide a better level of care?"

Then sit back and listen. These are some of the "pearls" that we have learned from dental sales "reps" in recent months:

- Laptop or I-pad in reception room for patients to submit positive reviews to Google Places.
- Ask each patient for a suggestion of one thing that could be done to improve the practice for them.
- Having patients' referrals enter them in a drawing for a monthly prize.
- Offer patients the ability to speak to satisfied patients who have had similar treatment to what we have presented to them.

Do not miss the opportunity to tap into the wealth of knowledge walking into our offices each and every day. Hand your "reps" a copy of this chapter and let them know this is what you will expect from them in the future for them to spend time with you.

CHAPTER 15

How To Hit Your Target

Howard Hill is considered the greatest archer of all time. He won 196 consecutive matches and he never lost in international competition. However, with that being said, I can boldly say that even with minimal training and practice, most of you could beat Howard Hill, on his very best day. The minor caveat here is that Howard Hill would be blindfolded and spun around a dozen times to destroy his sense of orientation. Many of you will laugh and say, "That's ridiculous! How can you hit a target you can't see?" Exactly! Many of you are, day in and day out, trying to hit goals that you don't have. You must have goals! Clearly constructed and defined goals!

For a goal to be effective it must effect change. Here are the steps in establishing goals for your practice:

1. Write your goals down.
2. Set a date.
3. Identify the obstacles.
4. Identify what you need to know.
5. Identify the people you need to work with

6.   Establish a plan
7.   Identify "What's in it for me?"

Figuratively, set long range goals as far as you can see and when you get there you will be able to see further. In 2007 when Peyton Manning won his first Super Bowl he was asked if it was the most thrilling achievement of his career. Without hesitating, he responded, "So far!" Do not let your accomplishments to be limited by past achievement or by underestimating your capabilities. Use the steps outlined above and take aim on your practice's bull's eye.

Category Three: People

CHAPTER 16

Follow The Yellow Brick Road
To Practice Growth

One of the most loved and classic movies of all time, "The Wizard of Oz", is celebrating its 75th Anniversary. The story describes how a young Kansas farm girl is whisked away by a "twister" to the Land of Oz. Accompanied by a knowledge-impaired Scarecrow, a caring-compromised Tin Man and a confidence-lacking Lion, Dorothy and her little dog, Toto, follow the Yellow Brick Road seeking the Wizard of Oz, in order that he might grant her wish to return home. The movie is full of symbolism and it is applicable to situations that we are experiencing in the field of dentistry.

Over the last few years we have witnessed numerous dental practices being whisked off track by the cumulative storm of poor economic conditions, commoditization and perceived constraints from horribly predatory insurance companies. This "twister" has been characterized by decreased new patient flow, fickle patients resisting treatment and a lack of depth in our schedules. As dentists have hopelessly spun in place they have seen opportunities and assurance that conditions would improve swirl out of reach. Barring further ineffectiveness by our government representatives failing to resolve the budget issues of our country, most practices have settled in at a new lower baseline. The hope is that the economic conditions that caused the storm have been eliminated, just as Dorothy's house settled on top of the Wicked Witch. Those who thought that hope was a strategy and that just tapping their mirrors and explorers together (instead of ruby slippers) would bring about change, might as well have been gazing over a rainbow:

Somewhere over the rainbow, way up high
There's a practice of dentistry I heard of once in a lullaby.
Somewhere over the rainbow, skies are blue.
And the dream that my practice can return to where it was can come true.
Somewhere over the rainbow, dentistry can become fulfilling with time
Practices are growing over the rainbow; why then oh why can't mine?

Others have been fortunate to have the voice of a Good Witch whispering in their ear that it is time to follow a Yellow Brick Road, of sorts, to redefine the vision of their practices and dedicate themselves to helping people improve their lives, to adopt more efficient systems and to invest in the development of their teams. Our Yellow Brick Road is paved with all of the building blocks of practice success. Without this type of plan and a dedication to working at these strategies, we might as well lay down in a field of poppies.

Dentists are like Dorothy. We are adept at looking around obstacles that inevitably appear in our paths. We have the need to gather a team to help us in our quest and once we have assembled this team we need to help them build their strengths and overcome any weaknesses. We must avoid the winged monkeys of gossip, negativity and selfishness to keep them focused on our Emerald City of practice success, financial and emotional fulfillment and personal satisfaction that exist at the end of the Yellow Brick Road.

So who comprise our partners on this road?

Our knowledge-impaired Scarecrows are our administrative teams. Most of them are prevented from performing at their highest level because dentists tend to micromanage and get in their way. We need to empower these team members, in particular. We must provide them with knowledge, resources and trust. When they possess these three building blocks they are equipped to take some winged monkeys off of our backs and to lessen the burden on Dorothy (dentists). The result is transforming straw-filled symbolic figures into confident, competent and resourceful managers for our practices.

Our caring-compromised Tin Men are our clinical assistants. In way too many practices we find that the criteria for selection of clinical assistants is based on clinical skills, relative cost and acceptable presentation. Those that excel in this role are the individuals who do have clinical experience and a clean and well-groomed appearance. However, of far more importance, are their core values and how much do they truly care about and relate to others. We must provide a caring and supportive environment for our team members so that they will, in turn, nurture the patients we serve. We must understand that those who can function in this way will have a greater self-worth and it would behoove dentists to recognize this dynamic and understand the need to compensate them accordingly.

Our confidence-lacking Lions may be our Hygienists. Most do NOT lack confidence, themselves, but where they lack confidence is in the knowledge of how much dentistry truly helps people to improve their lives. Many dentists and hygienists possess the same trait of approval addiction. We shy away from insisting that patients own their problems so as not to adversely affect their impression of us. Dentists and hygienists, both, must be confident in understanding the higher responsibility we have to affect people's lives, not just fix their teeth or heal their gums. Understand that we replace pain with comfort, that we help people enjoy life, that we eliminate poor self-esteem and build confidence, that we restore youth and enhance relationships and when our hygienists confidently own this ability they can roar like the King of the Jungle.

The Wicked Witches on our journey have been the dental insurance companies. Lowering benefits, regulating fees and limiting patients choices have created a situation where we must work twice or three times as hard as we once did to achieve the same return. If we don't find a way to neutralize the intentions of these insurance companies they will surely destroy all of us, "and our little dogs, too." We must adopt a strategy to inspire patients to seek care independent of their coverage. We must help them understand a compelling need to pursue our care. We must promote the benefits that we can provide so that dentistry moves up their list of priorities in establishing their discretionary budgets. If and when we accomplish this, our prowess will serve like the pail of water that Dorothy, the Scarecrow, the Tin Man and the Lion poured on the Witch's head and turned her into a heap of base plate wax.

We need to trust the instinctive abilities of the team members of our practices. As dental team members accept the responsibility to become more effective in promoting our practices and promoting the benefits that we provide for our patients, in helping to create a more positive culture within our practices and in maintaining an open mind to change for the better, then our offices will become, in a way, like Kansas and our practices will fulfill the prophecy that there is "no place like home".

CHAPTER 17

I Appreciate You!

M any dentists have a misconception of who the most important persons are in their practices. Some view themselves as being the only indispensable participant in the success of their practice, and in a pure sense, their assumption is valid. But in a much broader sense, this viewpoint is severely limited and limiting.

Others will insist that the patients come first and foremost. After all, they are our "raison d'etre" or our reason for being. Our practices are certainly dependent on our patients, but the quantity and quality of our patients can directly be attributed to the talents and capabilities of another group of individuals, the members of our teams.

The members of the team are, by far, the most important individuals in our practices. If you consider yourself successful as a practicing dentist, you certainly did not get there by yourself. (Didn't President Obama say that, as well?) When given adequate leadership, systems and resources, the team is in direct control of the practice potential. We have seen numerous superbly trained and talented dentists underachieving with a less than stellar team. Conversely, we have seen clinically challenged and socially uncomfortable doctors achieving phenomenal practice growth when surrounded by a strong team.

What do we need to do to enable our teams to drive our success? Get out of their way, stop micromanaging and encourage their decision-making. Show tolerance for errors since they are the source of greatest learning. And above all, show sincere appreciation.

Numerous sources indicate that the greatest motivator of employee performance is appreciation. Employers, such as dentists, commonly have the misconception that pay is the most important factor. However, as long as pay is fair and commensurate with skill and experience, team members are far more affected by sincere appreciation. One of the greatest complaints we hear from team members is that they receive little or no recognition or acknowledgement. Dentists who we've worked with will often hide behind excuses such as time or forgetfulness. Yet these same dentists will readily regurgitate complaints accumulated over a period of weeks. Those who say that they don't have the time to say "Thank you" for a job well done will have fewer opportunities as time progresses.

We recommend beginning each and every daily huddle, and certainly every team meeting, with acknowledgement of the positive things that team members have done the previous day or week. Always keep the acknowledgement completely positive. When there is anything contradictory to the compliment, save it for a different time and setting. Nothing should detract from the positivity of a direct and specific acknowledgement. Encourage team members to acknowledge each other. We have developed an "I Appreciate You" memo form for doctors and team members, alike, to use to acknowledge one another. These can be distributed at team meetings or given to the members of the team to present spontaneously, at will. They are simple, yet powerful, when used with total sincerity. We encourage you to use these forms. An image of the form can be seen below. If you would like to obtain padded copies of these forms please contact me at my email address, SmilePotential@aol.com.

I appreciate _____

because _____

_____

_____

Sincerely, _____

Smile Potential Dental Practice Coaching
Phone: 516-599-0214 / Email: SmilePotential@aol.com

CHAPTER 18

Tune Into Station WII-FM

Wherever we go today and whatever we do, we encounter people who have been victimized by lousy service and who are suspect of not being treated fairly. Trust, everywhere, has eroded and people generally walk around tuned into station WII-FM, where the question asked is "What's In It For Me?" The frequency of WII-FM is not necessarily bred from narcissism, but rather from the concern that life is more challenging today than it used to be and the choices we make should ultimately derive us some benefit.

People do not buy what we do or how we do it, but rather they buy in to the belief system of why we do it. Patients want to believe that we, their dentists, believe that we can make a difference in their lives. Therefore, when they ultimately make the decision to spend money on their dental care they want the confidence of knowing for sure that they are going to derive some benefit.

This is where the dis-connect exists which prevents many practices from being as successful as they can be. In dental school we were taught to explain the condition, offer a solution and describe the alternatives of care and the consequences of not receiving treatment. This strategy, while practical, will result in frequent refusal to pursue care. When dentists describe our procedures in technical minutiae, merely the names of our treatments conjure fearful images and association with negative consequences of treatment, such as discomfort and high cost. Even if we attempt to qualify our recommendations with describing the benefits, at this point, they go unheard because the patients remain fixated on all of the negativity implied by the description of the treatment.

If we choose to, instead, begin the conversation with a description of their problem and then list all of the benefits of treating that problem, this opens up an increased willingness in the patient to pursue treatment. Let's look at an example:

- Roger has a toothache. All clinical symptoms point to the need for a root canal. If we tell Roger he has an infection and that he needs a root canal, he will recall horror stories that he's heard about root canal treatment and make an assumption that it's very expensive. Even if we now describe the benefits of treatment, they will undoubtedly go unheard. However, if we begin by reinforcing the patient's ownership of his problem (the infection) and describe the consequences of not having treatment, it creates a "want" for the treatment that he needs. Next we should introduce the benefits of treatment, "In order to relieve your pain, enable you to retain the tooth for many years and restore the tooth with a beautiful, completely natural-looking restoration, we should begin by treating the tooth with a root canal." Emphasizing the benefits first increases the perceived value of the treatment, minimizes the concern for the previously described objections and greatly increases the likelihood of treatment acceptance. Station WII-FM is well tuned in at this point

This benefit-oriented approach should not be limited to just the description of treatment. I teach that the "New Patient Experience" should include a tour of the office. The tour should not merely be *"This is the sterilization area…and this is a treatment room…and this is our panorex…and this is the bathroom."* The scripting for the tour should be totally about benefits. Let the new "guest" to your office overdose on benefits. New patients are your best source of referrals. How different does it seem if you introduce the new patient to your practice this way?

- *"Welcome to our amazing practice. In order to make you feel at home we'd like to offer you a bottle of water, herbal tea or coffee before we begin a tour of our beautiful office. In order to provide you with the safest care available, we exceed all requirements for cleanliness and sterilization in this area…In order to provide you with the most up-to-date, state-of-the-art, hi-tech care we have (choose your technology, i.e. Digital x-ray, laser, Itero, etc.) here in our treatment room. In order to take your mind off of the treatment and keep you entertained we have ...(personal stereo, DVD movie collection, Live Mariachi Band, etc.). So that you may freshen up after we conclude your appointment we have lemon-scented hot towels, or here in the bathroom, we have scented lotions and hand creams. If there is anything else that we can do to make your experience a great one, just let us know."*

Don't you think this type of an introduction will add to the new patient's anticipation of a different and special experience? This type of introduction will increase the patient's "Wow" factor and ultimately make them more accepting of treatment.

Finally, no one listens more to station WII-FM than your team, and they absolutely should. In order to have a truly staff-driven practice, your team needs to be constantly reminded of the benefits of working in your office. When a team policy is changed, always present a benefit to THEM for the change. For example:

- With the rise in the cost of medical insurance it has been necessary for offices to cap the subsidized cost of coverage. One doctor we spoke with told his team that because of the increased premiums and leveling revenue, he could no longer afford to cover their insurance in full. What is the benefit to the team? Won't this breed resentment? Resentment leads to decreased motivation. However, if it were presented differently, it might actually serve to further motivate the team. *"It is my intention to provide all of you with an increasingly generous benefits package. Recent circumstances have increased the financial burden on the practice. In order to insure the security of all of your positions and to enable me to continue all of you having medical coverage it will become necessary to have everyone assume a minimal share in the expense. As soon as all of you help the practice overcome this challenge we will be able to reverse this decision. Can I count on your cooperation to work together to get this behind us?"*

Which approach will achieve a better response to a lousy situation? Everyone we deal with each and every day in our practice is motivated by the same basic instincts, desire for pleasure and avoidance of pain. Our verbal skills have as much to do with satisfying these instincts as anything we can do. Always take the time to consider refined ways of describing why you do what you do. Then and only then will those around you be interested in what you do or how you do it. Tune in to station WII-FM and watch your listening audience grow.

CHAPTER 19

Savor The Relationships

I found the headline, "The End of the Doctor-Patient Relationship," in an April, 2013 edition of Newsweek to be very upsetting. What has become of our professions? If relationships are not strong in something as personalized as medical and dental care, then the level of care is bound to suffer. In a survey by Consumer Reports, 70% of health care professionals reported that since they began practicing, the bond with their patients has eroded. Concurrently, studies show a steep decline over the last three decades in patients' sense of satisfaction and the feeling that they are receiving high-quality care. Dr. Howard Brody, Director of the Institute for Medical Humanity, has written, "There is something in the human body that says we are hardwired to get better when we have a certain relationship with the person treating us." Numerous studies have also shown that there is a link between how well the doctor and patient communicate and the patient's sense of wellbeing, number of symptoms and overall health.

With that being said, I want every dentist, hygienist, clinical assistant and administrative team member to make a firm commitment to changing the paradigm and dedicating their efforts to reestablishing strong relationships with all of your patients. I will emphatically state that this is the single most important thing that you can due to insure the success of your practices and to finding fulfillment in your chosen field.

The relationship is important because it is the vehicle by which we establish believability, likability and trust. The longer it takes to develop a relationship the longer it takes to develop the confidence that allows us to enlist patients in care which will benefit them most.

The relationship should begin well before the patient ever enters the office. Those who answer the phones should speak with a friendly tone and use value-adding language. A good closing for the initial phone call is to say, *"My job is to help make your experience in our office a positive one."*

Often times, new patients will fail to present for their initial appointment. The reason this occurs is that they have no connection to the doctor or their team. The recommendation that I make to our clients is for the DOCTOR to call all scheduled first-time patients the night before their first visit. Whether you reach the patient, or their voicemail, the script should read something like, *"Hello Mr. / Mrs. New Patient. This is Dr. Wonderful, the dentist who you will be visiting with tomorrow. I like to call the night before our first meeting to welcome you to the practice, to introduce myself and find out if there are any particular concerns that you have before you come in. I very much look forward to meeting you and to caring for you and your family for many years to come."* Whether or not you actually speak to the patient or leave this message on their voicemail, they will all mention that they have never received a phone call like that before. Do you think that may contribute to a different type of doctor/patient relationship?

When the "new" patient presents to the office for the first time they should not be treated like a patient, but more like a special visitor to your home. This forbids sliding a glass window open and handing them a clip-board. This means coming out from behind the admin-istrative desk and greeting them by name with a two-handed handshake. The next step is to help them off with their coat, offer refreshments and take them on a benefit-oriented tour of your office. If they have not already completed the registration forms, they should be made comfortable in a private consultation room so that they can complete the forms comfortably on a desk instead of leaning into their lap, concerned that some-one might see their information.

Relationship building continues when a member of the team sits with the patient inquiring about past dental experiences and identifying their expectations of care. Then the doctor is introduced to the patient and he or she spends time eye-to-eye in this non-clinical setting getting to know the patient. Before any clinical discus-sion it is important to find out about their family, their occupation, recent and upcoming personal milestones and finally what prompted them to present to the dental practice. In dental school we are all trained to identify the "Chief Complaint" or condition that exists. The truth is that the patient doesn't really care about that condition. They are more concerned about how that condition affects their life. If we can tap into the emotional "disability" caused by the "condition" we have a much stronger likelihood that the patient will accept the treatment we design to correct this disability. The reason for this success in treatment acceptance is directly related to the strength of the relationship that is created through the practices previously described.

Additional strategies to reinforce the relationship include respecting patients time by starting out on time (SOOT), staying on time (SOT) and getting out on time (GOOT). SOOT/SOT/GOOT is one of the biggest practice builders that we can practice. I recommend the doctor calling patients who receives anesthetic for a procedure in the evening, after their appointment. This, too, will differentiate you from all dentists they have been to previously.

The bottom line is that anything we do to build and reinforce the relationship with our patients will ultimately raise the perceived value of receiving care in your office. When the perceived value goes up, the perceived cost of care goes down, in the patients mind. And when this occurs, patients are much more likely to agree to treatment, and certainly more comprehensive and cosmetic treatment, independent of insurance benefits. In addition, it is well established that the stronger relationship will increase the level of satisfaction with the level of care received. What could be better? Savor the relationship.

CHAPTER 20

Pearls From 3 Unlikely Sources

When I began coaching and consulting with dental practices five years ago I was confident that I had a wealth of knowledge that I could impart to my dental colleagues that would help them improve their performance within their practices. I am proud of what Kelly Fox-Galvagni and I have achieved in working with dozens of dentists and their teams throughout the New York metropolitan area. We have seen several practices double their production and profitability. We have helped numerous practices implement systems that have enabled them to achieve new highs in treatment acceptance and patient satisfaction while drastically decreasing the amount of stress they deal with on a daily basis. We have facilitated the development of teamwork and positive practice cultures that have transformed our clients' practice environments to where each member of the team relishes the opportunity to work in such a fun, cooperative and rewarding atmosphere and where motivation has become second nature. These were components of the vision that Kelly and I set out with in 2009. But now as we try to evaluate our performance and redefine our vision we are finding that our original vision was flawed. Neither of us ever accounted for how much we would learn in the process of trying to teach others. We learn a tremendous amount from each of the practices that we work with. Much of what we learn from one practice we are then able to cross-pollinate into the other practices each and every month.

Furthermore, I have learned a tremendous amount in the preparation for presentations and speaking engagements and in the development of agendas for our numerous team meetings each month. It is astounding how much I am learning from individuals outside the field of dentistry. While dentistry is a unique field with numerous idiosyncrasies, it is also so similar to many other service industries.

The first unlikely "mentor" that I will reference in this chapter is an individual who has mastered the strategies needed to motivate clients to accept and want elective care. Most books and videos about sales deal with the mechanics of selling, and while this is important, it does not touch on the strong emotional component of the process. One of the gurus of sales and marketing is Dan Kennedy. Dan Kennedy coauthored a book, "Uncensored Sales Strategies", with Sydney Biddle Barrows, the Mayflower Madam. In this book they discuss selling your customers (or patients) what they really want. By understanding that our patients are not buying teeth any more than Ms. Barrows clients were buying sex, we learn that we have the ability to fulfill patients' fantasies. Each and every patient that wants cosmetic dentistry is really looking to fulfill a fantasy that they are a celebrity or a movie star with a dazzling smile that is just one component of an enhanced presentation. Furthermore, these patients are very much seduced by the experience. Understand that patients will prefer to be cared for by someone that they have a relationship with; individuals they know, like and trust and who they feel know and like them. This is why we need to spend as much time getting to know as much about our patients as we can before they ever sit back in our chairs and open their mouths. We need to not only inquire about the nature of their dental concerns, but we need to focus more on how these concerns impact on their lives. Does the dental "condition" create a feeling of embarrassment, interference in concentration or a disruption of function? These are the disabilities that patients want to disengage from, not the chip, fracture or discoloration that we tend to focus on in our typical blinder-hindered perspective. Remove the blinders and begin focusing on the human aspect of dental care. Then realize that you can position yourself ahead of the crowd by creating an experience in your office that is memorable in a positive way. Be creative because the quality of the experience can significantly add to the perceived value of the service you provide. The general nature of the baby boomers, which seek the highest percentage of our elective care, is that they will pay more for a service if it is delivered with an experience that is pleasurable and meaningful to them. Dental patients are consumers who are bored with uniformity and associate it with mediocrity. Your vision needs to incorporate the creation of an interesting and exciting environment that supports the nurturing connection you will be making with your patients on an emotional level.

This leads in to the second "mentor" from this trio. Johnny is a 19-year-old "bagger" in a Midwestern supermarket. Johnny has Down's syndrome. When Johnny's boss asked each of his employees to do something to benefit his store, most of his employees responded with typical pledges to come in on time, improve their personal grooming, maintain store cleanliness and be more courteous to customers. Johnny couldn't think of anything concrete but he went home and saw that his calendar had a thought for each day. Johnny's idea was to come up with a thought for each of his customers. He began to think of a kind thought each day. One day it was, "Today I will give you a big smile. Will you smile back to me?" The next day it was, "Today was a beautiful day because we said hello to each other". Each day he thought of a simple idea and had his Dad type it on the computer and print 500 copies of the thought. Johnny would then cut the sayings into strips of paper and place them on the top of each customer's groceries with a sincere "Have a nice day!" Before long, the line at Johnny's register became consistently longer than at any of the other registers. Some customers started coming in multiple times each week just to get Johnny's thought for the day. Sometimes they brought friends and neighbors. Johnny's "Thought for the Day" fueled an incredible increase in business for the supermarket. Who on each of your teams has the ability to think outside the box to create a special environment within your practices? Who will become your Johnny? Give your teams the opportunity to be creative and reward their inventiveness.

This leads into the final "mentor" of this group. Nick Vujicic is a 29-year-old young man who was born in Australia without arms or legs. Yet, Nick has become a well-educated motivational speaker. He has transformed his short life without limbs to accomplish more than most other individuals will ever achieve in a lifetime. He has founded a worldwide organization called "Life Without Limits". He is an incredible motivational speaker who inspires others to draw strength from the challenges they face. In a video of one speech, Nick can be seen laying face down, flat on his stomach. He talks about how difficult it is for him to get up and how he may try 100 times and not be able to become upright. He asks the question that if he gives up will he EVER get up? The answer is a resounding "NO". But, if he continues to persevere, no matter how exhausted he is, he WILL eventually get up and he does accomplish that feat with much effort. The message to "Never Give Up" applies to us in each of our practices. In these challenging times we must creatively search for new ways to attract patients and to enhance the patient experience. Some of the ideas will not work. Other ideas may have limited success. But eventually, if we never give up, we

will persevere and find ways in which we can impact on
the success of our practices now and for the future.

Thus, the challenge we all face, as demonstrated by
these three very unlikely sources is to realize the importance of relationships and the experience within our
practices. Then to search for creative ways to make the
experience so positive that our patients would never
think of going anywhere else and to make a commitment to keep trying new and inventive ideas and to
never give up until we find ideas that work for us in our
own situations.

CHAPTER 21

A Lesson From The Monkey Cage

All too often when we visit practices we find doctors and their teams performing tasks without much of a sense of commitment. They tend to be going through the motions. When questioned, they also lack a sense of purpose or of understanding as to why they are doing the tasks the way that they are. One of the best examples of this is that many doctors routinely make hygienists and their patients wait for them to perform their perfunctory "check". This results in frustration on the part of the hygienist, resentment on the part of the waiting patient and disappointment on the part of the delayed succeeding hygiene patient. When asked why doctors wait until the end of the hygiene appointment to do the check, in spite of the fact that there might have been a more efficient time, they usually refer to the fact that "they've always done it this way". The same can be said for teams who wipe down their counters with alcohol, for doctors who routinely perform root canals over the course of multiple appointments and administrative teams who file for insurance predeterminations for preventive treatment. When questioned about why these tasks were performed in certain ways, the response is always that "we've always done it that way".

Recently, one of my daughters was taking a course in Human Development. In her textbook there was the story of an experiment involving five monkeys that could be applied to this phenomenon. A scientist, according to the story, did an experiment with five monkeys housed in a cage. The scientist hung a bunch of bananas in the cage where the monkeys could not reach them. A large tree branch was put up against the wall close to the bananas. One monkey figured out that he could climb the branch and reach the bananas. But just as he was about to grab them, the scientist used a hose and drenched all the monkeys with cold, frigid water and chaos ensued. Later another of the monkeys tried to get the bananas and again the scientist drenched them with the ice-cold water. This occurred several more times until one of the monkeys made the connection between reaching for the bananas and the cold water.

On the next attempt, that monkey attacked the one who was trying to get the bananas and prevented him from doing so. The others joined in when it became clear that reaching for the bananas caused the water punishment to start. After that, none of the monkeys tried to get the bananas.

Later, the scientist took out one of the monkeys and included a new one. The new monkey saw the bananas and tried to reach them. The original four monkeys attacked the newcomer when it made its attempt. They managed to stop him before the water punishment started. This monkey also learned not to try to get the bananas. The scientist then removed another of the original monkeys and included a new one. The process was repeated and eventually the new monkey would join in the attack, even though it did not know why.

The scientist removed the original monkeys one by one, replacing them with a new monkey each time. Each time the reaction was the same. The new monkey was attacked when it tried to get the bananas. Eventually, all of the original monkeys had been replaced. All this time none of the new monkeys had ever been sprayed with water. Even though they did not know why, all of the replacement monkeys kept attacking the new monkey every time they tried to get the bananas.

Why did this happen? All of the new monkeys had learned "That's how we do things around here. That's how it's always been done." Does this sound like anything in your practices? Systems need to constantly be reviewed for efficiency and relevancy. It is important to confirm why we do things the way that we do them. There may have been a good reason to do something a certain way a long time ago, but it may not be applicable now. Always be open to new ideas, new strategies, new techniques and new technologies. Get the monkeys off your back and you may find that there are better, more efficient and more cost effective ways of performing tasks and procedures. Some of these ideas may rattle your cage, for a while, but in time you will find that the bananas previously out of reach will afford you the ability to make banana splits, banana daiquiris, bananas foster and they may offer many other advantages that you may never have realized previously. Quit monkeying around!

CHAPTER 22

Write Your Own "50 Shades Of Grey"

One of the most popular books of recent years was "50 Shades of Grey" by E.L. James. It described a perverse relationship, deeply rooted in abuse and domination. It was such a steamy book that few people would read it with the cover in view of others. Its sales exploded in the e-book market where confidentiality in reading choices could be maintained, had it not been for the gaping looks and sweaty brows caused by the content of the story. No book read mostly by women, craving the lust of a romance novel, had ever been borrowed by spouses and significant others as much as "50 Shades of Grey". It ignited a new sexual revolution of sorts.

Our practices are also in need of something revolutionary. What is going on in many practices is also perverse and a threat to healthy relationships. It threatens the emotional health of practices and it leaves team members exasperated with frustration. But before you get all hot and bothered, I want to affirm that it has nothing to do with sex, though it may touch on abuse and domination, of a different sort and it can be emotionally scarring. It has to do with all of the "stuff" that clouds our sense of purpose in the daily delivery of care and caring.

The root of the problem is undefined expectations of others. Most of the expectations of doctors for their team members can be described as black, or white. "I expect her to be on time." "I expect them to clean up the staff room after lunch." "I expect her to be prepared for the team meeting." "I expect the reception room to be vacuumed before we leave for the evening." "I can't believe why she doesn't get it!"

The problem with these expectations is not that they exist, but that they have not been clearly defined for the team members involved. The team members may be thinking, "It doesn't matter if I get there a few minutes late. The doctor doesn't stroll in until a quarter past." "I'll leave it for Mary to clean up because I cleaned up after lunch last Tuesday." "What can I contribute to the meeting? I'm just an assistant." "What difference does it make if I vacuum tonight or if I come in 15 minutes early in the morning?" "I don't know what the doctor expects of me!"

All of these are "grey" areas. In the absence of some clearly defined determination of what is expected, it can be up for interpretation. This is why we recommend that each practice generate its own "50 Shades of Grey" or a "Culture Guide", of sorts, to clearly define the expectations, in writing, for every member of the team. These expectations should be written and placed in a "Culture Guide" binder to be kept in full access to all of the team.

Some of the areas that can be addressed in this guide would be punctuality, expected levels of preparation for meetings and huddles, defining housekeeping responsibilities, determining the expected tone for interactions with patients and fellow team members, orchestrating teamwork for rotated responsibilities, expressing the importance of coordination for emergency or extended scheduling challenges, or anything similar. When these responsibilities are clearly defined and each team member receives a copy, then there is no longer confusion over the "grayness" of expectations. When expectations are clearly defined, then performance can be accurately evaluated and when appropriate, rewarded or questioned. When these "gray zones" are eliminated, so are the arguments, hard feelings and disappointments that go along with them and there is much greater harmony in the practice.

We encourage you to schedule a team meeting to identify some of the "Grey" areas in your practices. Engage in respectful discussion. Come to definitive decisions. Try to have fun with it and be creative. But please leave the feathers, whips, handcuffs and blindfolds home…that day.

CHAPTER 23

No More "Butt-Dialing"

We have all had the experience of picking up a ringing phone and hearing at the other end either laughter, a random conversation or something that was not intended for our ears. The fact is that we have been "butt-dialed" on a phone in someone's pocket. There are documented stories of "butt-dialing" in the midst of trysts, which have alerted previously unsuspecting partners.

The fact of the matter is that there is also rampant "butt-dialing" going on in the hallways of our dental practices. On a recent practice observation I was in a treatment room reviewing the practice's schedule and management reports on one of the operatory computers when I heard in the hallway three different "butt-dialing" conversations. The first was describing how bad the breath was of Mr. Violated, who was sitting in the hygienist's chair at that very moment. The second was of the hygienist stating how much she drank the night before. The third was of an assistant describing the dentist as a "jerk" because he kept her 20 minutes late the previous evening while treating an emergency and then he had the nerve to say something about her gum chewing in the office.

Because our patients are in a somewhat threatening environment in our treatment rooms, their sensory awareness is at a heightened state. They hear everything that we say within earshot and some of the conversations in the hallways outside our treatment rooms do not paint our practices in a positive light. Our teams must avoid speaking about patients, especially when it is negative gossip. They must avoid speaking about their own behaviors, which may be misconstrued (or not) to affect their job performance. They must avoid speaking unfavorably about any other member of the dental team. When patients hear these conversations it causes them to lose confidence in our care. When they lose confidence in our care they tend to accept less dental care from us. We must limit our conversations in patient earshot to only positive discussions that show we care deeply about our patients and about each other. When patients hear conversations like this it enhances their opinion of the culture in our office and of those about to render them care. This makes them far more accepting of the type of care we would like to provide.

CHAPTER 24

The Less Patients Feel,
The More Positive They Will Feel About You

Wherever we go to speak to dentists we are asked for strategies to grow practices, increase case acceptance and improve referrals. The answer to all three of these challenges was taught to us as one of the most basic clinical skills in dental school. The extent to which we strive to perfect that skill is one of the most important keys to the success of our practices.

It is impossible to understate the importance of giving effective and absolutely painless anesthetic injections. The key to a painless injection begins long before the needle penetrates tissue and absolutely involves the participation of the entire team. Do not underestimate the importance of the team's verbal skills in helping the patient to formulate the expectation of a painless injection.

This expectation raises the patient's confidence and lowers the anticipation of a painful experience. In sports this concept is called visualization. Visualization is the exercise of seeing oneself go through a task or performance prior to actually experiencing it. In the process of visualization an athlete virtually experiences success prior to actually achieving it. In our practices, the level of compassion shown by the team has a similar effect on the patient seeing them self have a positive injection experience.

Compassion is the most important quality that we can possess. A total realization that we can absolutely make a difference in whether our patient suffers through the injection is more important than any physical thing we do. With that being said, I will pass on some of the things that we have found in our practice to provide our patients with totally comfortable care.

1. Use the most effective topical anesthetic available. There are numerous "topicals" available in our dental catalogues and at dental meetings, but the most effective one that we have found is PFG gel, formerly "Profound", formulated by Steven's Pharmacy in Costa Mesa, California. PFG contains a combination of tetracaine, lidocaine and prilocaine. Apply it for a sufficient amount of time and your patients will not feel your injections. For more information about PFG, you may look them up at www.stevensrx.com.

2. Have your clinical assistant massage the shoulder of your patient beginning just before you deliver your injection. I don't mean a light tap. I mean a serious massage of the shoulder and

upper arm. It is comforting and it is also a diversion. Whatever the mechanism, it gives the patient the feeling that you and your team care and it symbolizes "hands-on" healing and promotes confidence.

3. View Dr. Jeffrey Hoos' video, *"Now You Can Get Painless, Profound, Predictable Anesthesia Without Topical, The Wand or Vibra Jet"*. It is the best instructional video I have ever seen about administering anesthetic injections. It is available through www.theprofitabledentist.com.

4. Administer your injections as slow as you possibly can. Be sure you stretch unattached tissue at the site of puncture to minimize the trauma of penetration and then wait a sufficient amount of time for it to become maximally effective. For mandibular block injections I recommend waiting a minimum of 10 minutes…but DO NOT run out of the treatment room and leave the patient alone. Use this time for reinforcing the relationship between you and the patient. Use the time to talk about innovations in your practice. Use it to discuss your beliefs and let them know why being a dentist excites you. Remember that people do not buy how or what you do, but instead they buy why you do it.

5. Make sure your anesthesia is sufficiently profound for the procedure that you are performing. It doesn't matter how painless your injection is if

the patient continues to feel pain. Test the sight and stop immediately to re-inject if the patient shows any sign of feeling even the slightest discomfort. Never minimize what the patient is feeling and never ask or expect them to tolerate discomfort. Remember there is an increasingly positive progression of how a patient can describe an experience in your practice; very bad, bad, o.k., good and great. Only great matters. Only great inspires people to change their habits and try a "new" dentist.

6. In spite of what Dr. Hoos' says in his DVD, consider using the "Wand", which is a computerized delivery system for anesthetic. In our practice, we have found the "Wand" to be of great value in delivering comfortable anesthesia to multiple sites. There are many positives about the "Wand" including comfort, lack of regional numbness, and the perceived value of the more advanced technology. It is also wonderful for the treatment of children. For more information about the Wand, look at www.milestonescientific.com.

7. We have had tremendous success in our practice in using Dental Vibe to reduce patient anxiety by eliminating injection pain. The Dental Vibe is a cordless, rechargeable device that delivers soothing, pulsed oscillations to the

injection site while the injection is being administered. It stimulates the sensory receptors in the area and interferes with the body's ability to detect discomfort. The Dental Vibe is a relatively inexpensive instrument that is well received by the patients and it has been universally successful in every region of the mouth. For more information go to www.DentalVibe.com. I have spoken to Dr. Steven Goldberg, the inventor and CEO of Dental Vibe and he has agreed to extend a discount to anyone mentioning Smile Potential and using the promo code "KATZ".

8. Consider using an anesthetic reversal agent for procedures not expected to give post-operative pain. Patients often complain of the duration of anesthesia, almost as much as about receiving the anesthesia in the first place. Oraverse (phentolamine mesylate) is the first medication available to decrease the duration of numbness through injection at the same site as the original injection. Oraverse is a costly medication to administer, but it is also a value-adding service for patients needing to return to work or a social engagement following treatment. It is a wonderful adjunct for children to avoid the secondary trauma of cheek, lip or tongue biting as a result of being numb.

When you master the technique for delivering painless, effective injections it benefits your practice on many levels. Patients who have a painless injection experience have a higher level of confidence. This makes them much more likely to accept elective cosmetic treatment and more comprehensive care.

Everything we do within our practices is marketing. When your patients have a positive experience, such as a painless injection and a pain free procedure, they are far more likely to tell others. Our patients are not interested in the tertiary anatomy in a posterior restoration. In their minds the measure of whether we are a good dentist, or not, is whether we give a painless injection. We do not get a second chance to make a good first impression. When they comment to any member of our team, it creates an opportunity for us to acknowledge their positive experience, to reassert the practice's dedication to totally comfortable care and to directly ask for referrals. Take advantage of those opportunities and you will see your reputation improve and your practice continue to grow.

CHAPTER 25

It's Not About The Money

This may seem to be a strange topic for a Practice Management Coach to be writing about. In April, 2013 our dental practice, Smiles On Broadway, had a wonderful party at our office for patients, neighbors, colleagues and dental vendors to celebrate that we had been voted "The Best Dental Practice On Long Island for 2013" in the Long Island Press. I want to emphasize the fact that I am <u>NOT</u> the best dentist on Long Island, though I believe that I am extremely talented and dedicated to excellence in care. I don't know who the best dentist is. I have seen exquisite cosmetic dentistry performed by many well-trained dentists in our backyard, some trained at LVI and other institutes. I have sat in awe of the knowledge about occlusion and function practiced by graduates of Dawson, Pankey and similar dental brain trusts. I have seen procedures performed by Oral Surgeons, Periodontists, Endodontists and Orthodontists right here on Long Island that border on the miraculous and are testimonials to the possibilities that we can create in dentistry today. While I will assert that quality of care is of the paramount importance in our practice and I perform dentistry to the best of my ability on <u>every</u> single patient each and <u>every</u> day and that I am <u>constantly</u> seeking to <u>improve</u> through continuing education, the one and only reason that we have been voted "Best" is that we provide our patients with the best experience that they could ever imagine in a professional office and they have shown their appreciation by casting those votes. Our patients, your patients, have no sense of clarity in what "quality dentistry" is. They can look in the mirror and see dentistry that looks good to them, but they will not be able to see open margins, or missed decay that might come back to haunt them later. They have no way of gauging what they can't see. What they care about is whether they <u>Believe</u> we are doing the right thing, do they <u>Like</u> us, and do they <u>Trust</u> us. The diet for success in our practices is this very "B L T" sandwich. Maya Angelou, the great poet, once said, *"People will forget what you said, they will forget what you did, but they will never forget how you made them feel."* Show them you care because patients will not care about how much you know until they know how much you care.

As we've mentioned previously, the basis for making our patients feel one way or another has nothing to do with what we do or how we do it. For the most part, all of us in our practices do basically the same things using similar techniques, materials, labs and philosophies. Our patients derive their inspiration to come to us, or stay with us based on a belief that we can help them. The purpose that we have developed for our practice, and it is my own personal purpose, as well, is

"To make a difference in people's lives." Isn't that what we do, however we do it, when we relieve pain, transform appearances and improve the quality of life the way we do? You better believe it is.

When you practice with this sense of purpose, you also encounter situations that, ultimately, make a difference in your own life. Every dentist I speak to can relate at least one story where, out of kindness or generosity that they have impacted on a patient's life and reciprocally felt fulfilled from the effort.

There are two patient situations that come to mind in our practice. Paul has been a union member with "local" insurance coverage. Every time his wife and family came to our office for treatment he would complain about the fees and the lack of coverage his insurance provided in our office. After many years, one of his daughters required extensive emergency care. Against his wife and daughter's outrage, he insisted that his daughter go to the "plan" provider. After only one visit there, however, Paul returned to our practice, and deeply apologized for whatever he had said previously. He expressed appreciation for the level of care and caring we provided his family. Paul has since had extensive treatment done in our practice, himself, and has been one of our most supportive patients and best sources of referrals. While I can insist till I'm blue in the face that I made a difference for Paul, really he affected me much more by validating the way we care for our patients.

Jeannette is a wonderful woman who lost a child to cancer two years ago, after a protracted and costly course of treatment, which exhausted her life savings. The care of her son limited her to emergency visits in our office. Our entire team thought it would be nice to provide free care to Jeannette to enhance her smile so she could smile at her son through his illness. Unfortunately, her son passed away soon after we began her treatment. Not long after the death of her son, "Superstorm Sandy" destroyed Jeannette's home, and she, additionally, lost both of her cars. She considered our practice her sanctuary. Our team decided that smile enhancement was not enough for Jeannette, so we redeveloped her plan into a full-mouth reconstruction, including extensive bone grafting, implants, implant-supported fixed prosthetics and exquisite porcelain veneers. The treatment has most definitely improved our patient's state of mind. It has given her the self-esteem to reenter the world around her with confidence and she is establishing a new purpose for her life. When we completed her care we were enveloped in a feeling of tremendous accomplishment. Through the course of Jeannette's care, her appointments were among our most anticipated. No appointments were more satisfying and gratifying to provide. No treatment we have ever done has ever been more appreciated.

As previously mentioned, our purpose is "To make a difference in people's lives". We have certainly brought change and improvement to Paul and Jeannette's lives.

There is a tremendous level of poignancy; however, when we look deeper and realize the tremendous benefit that we have derived from these efforts. Sure, we've gotten some referrals, but more importantly we have realized the full potential of how we have the ability to change lives and not just fix teeth and treat gums. Develop a sense of purpose in your practices that refocuses the goals of you and your team to exceed, on various levels, what you do and how you do it.

CHAPTER 26

Keep It Real

A friend of mine is a skier. During a trip last winter to Vail, he found himself on a chair lift with a snowboarder. In the world of downhill winter sports there is a schism that exists between skiers and snow-boarders. They are wildly different styles competing for space on the hill. The rivalry seems to bring out a level of obnoxiousness when in the company of the other "camp". The boarder began the conversation with *"Wha's up, Dude?"* At that moment my friend's inner BS generator went into hyper drive and this Brooklyn-born "deese, dats and dose" kind of guy, who failed level one French in middle school, answered in a perfect French accent, "Sacre bleu!"

The conversation went like this:

Snowboarder: *"Dude, this is a most excellent day. Are you shredding?"*

My friend: *"Eet iz une day terrifique!*

Snowboarder: *"Are you from France?"*

Friend: *"Oui!"*

Snowboarder: …Well, it doesn't even pay to recount the string of sentences the young Frenchmen began cascading, in perfect French, having been born and raised in Albertville, in the French Alps. My friend had no choice but to come clean and make a rapid exit from the lift with his tail between his snow pants. To this day, he refuses to ever meet for dinner in a French restaurant.

We talk a lot about "Integrity" in business. Dentistry is a profession deeply rooted in trust and integrity. It's hard to measure, but the concept is so simple and succinct. If you know what's right, do what's right. Choose rightness over ease and convenience. Do not succumb to compromise when faced with challenges. In the words of Martin Luther King Jr., *"The ultimate measure of a man is not where he stands in moments of comfort and convenience, but where he stands at times of challenge and controversy."*

In the past year I have encountered several upsetting scenarios. In an initial interview with a potential client, I asked him to describe his practice. His wife chimed in with "My husband runs a QUALITY practice. He does GORGEOUS work! Just look at what he did for me." Then she lifted up her lip to show the most hideous anterior bridge we have ever seen, refrigerator-white horse-teeth with thick black margins far from fire-engine-red swollen gums. During a subsequent observation we found his lab work was sent to China for $49/unit, he re-used disposable products and washed his gloves between patients.

A second scenario involves a dentist, who touts what a high quality practice he has. When an assistant from one of our client's practices "temped" for him a while back she reported that he had instructed her to "not put the handpieces in the autoclave because it destroys the turbines." Instead he told her to seal the handpieces in sterilizer pouches so that he could open them in front of his patients and they would see the illusion that they were sterilized.

There are three components to anyone's personality. They are:

1. How you want to be perceived
2. How you perceive yourself
3. How you truly are

Until these three distinct perspectives are brought into harmony there is a failure in our ability to act and perform with integrity. We understand that times may be more difficult, on several planes, but the need to do everything possible to maintain trust is paramount in what we do. We all like to think that we are one way or another and we like to think that others perceive us in that same way. The true test of our integrity is if we act that way when no one is holding us accountable. This is when we show our true nature.

In these times it is important to advocate for our practices. We must paint our practices in the best light possible so that we can attract new patients eager to receive our care. Based on how we market our practices, patients come to us with preconceived expectations. If you fail to meet these expectations, they will likely move on to another practice. Thus, it becomes necessary for us to constantly exceed expectations. When you exceed the expectations of those who you serve, they will do the bragging for you. If you are going to "Talk the talk" you better damn well make sure that you "Walk the walk."

The lesson for the business of our dental practices, as well as in life is, "if you don't speak the language, don't fake the accent." Or, in the words of your average snowboarder, "Keep it real!"

CHAPTER 27

A Lesson From My Daughter

One of he events I look forward to each year is the Greater New York Dental Meeting. It begins over Thanksgiving weekend at the Jacob Javits Convention Center on the west side of Manhattan. This year as I attended lectures and walked the aisles of the exhibit floor I was struck by the predominance of dentists and team members looking for solutions to problems. The problem of the economy, the problem of low new patient numbers, the problem of decreased production and lower income, the problem of low staff motivation, and the problem of open time in the schedule.... these were among the problems that attendees were looking to solve.

My other, and more important, pursuit of the Thanksgiving holiday weekend is spending time with my family. As my daughters have entered adulthood, it is not often that the five of us get to spend quality time together merely enjoying each other's company.

A business lesson from the holiday weekend a couple of years ago came from my eldest daughter, Heather. After she graduated from the Newhouse School at Syracuse University she accepted an internship in "web project management" for a startup Internet

Company called Betterfly.com. As her position evolved into gainful and fulfilling employment, I was more than a casual observer of the prospects for success of this company. The premise of Betterfly.com was that we, as people, are our own biggest asset, and therefore we should invest in ourselves and become better. Betterfly.com was an online service that connected people with mentors, coaches, tutors, and trainers etc.… What we need in dentistry is the philosophy of Betterfly.com. We must start looking to the future and how we can improve ourselves, patient relationships, our team relationships, our clinical skill sets, our communication skills, our level of organization and business prowess. Forget the problems that have been bogging us down. Most of these problems have been out of our control anyway. Let's focus on improvement in the areas where we can exert some level of personal control. If we can make strides in the improvement of some of these areas, success of our practices will inevitably follow. How can we initiate this process?

My recommendation is to schedule a full day for a team meeting. It is an opportunity to redefine the Vision for your practice and develop an Action Plan for the success in attaining your vision. During the course of this day you and your teams will identify goals, establish timetables, create a budget, anticipate obstacles and restructure job descriptions in congruence with the practice vision. Where will the ideas come from?

I strongly recommend that each and every one of you acquire a book entitled "I-Power" by Martin Edelstein. "I-Power" describes a practical system for brainstorming. It shows how to encourage every member of your team to think about how each of them works and encourages them to contribute Information and Ideas on how to do everything better. A meeting based on "I-Power" will result in Ideas, Ingenuity, Incentives, Individual achievement, Invigorating concepts, Inquisitiveness into processes, Innovation, Inspiration, Imagination and, ultimately, Improvement. We must redirect out attention from solving past problems to searching for ways to develop improvement.

CHAPTER 28

The Lesson Of The 5 Balls

In his commencement speech to the graduating class of Georgia Tech University in 1991, Bryan Dyson, the CEO of Coca Cola, spoke about the *"Lesson of the Five Balls"*. The story was popularized 15 years later in a sappy novel by James Patterson entitled *"Suzanne's Diary for Nicholas"*.

Imagine life is a game in which you are juggling five balls in the air. You name them – Work – Family – Health – Friends – Integrity. The five balls pretty much sum up what's important in life and your goal is to keep all of them within your control. You should understand that one of the balls, Work, is made of rubber. It is flexible and it can reliably rebound. This is not the case with the other four balls, which are made of glass. If you drop any one of the other balls, Family – Health – Friends or Integrity, they may become irreversibly scuffed, marked, damaged, or even shattered. They will never be the same. These balls must be juggled with care, gentleness and purpose and this is how we must strive for balance in our lives.

During the first 15 years of my dental career I was a workaholic. When I was in my "work mode" almost nothing could derail me. My absolute priority was growing my practice to achieve the dream of my vision. Success fueled even greater effort until, in 1998, I was mistakenly diagnosed with Colon Cancer. A series of innocent diagnostic errors, in combination, led a prominent Gastroenterologist to a premature erroneous conclusion. His exact words to my wife and I that Friday afternoon were, "We've discovered a mass in your colon which seems to be malignant. I have scheduled you for further tests in the hospital on Tuesday. As you can see, I'm very busy. If you have any further questions, speak to my secretary". And then he left the room. I will spare comment on the lack of this doctor's professionalism and sensitivity. In retrospect, I think he was an anal orifice (AO). But I can tell you how he instilled in me a level of fear, initially, and regret, secondarily. I feared for my life and for all that I stood to miss if the disease were to get the best of me. I regretted that I had failed to fully embrace other aspects of my life, family and friends, and all of the joys that can be derived from them. I spent the weekend changing light bulbs and installing the paper towel dispenser that had been in a box for several months. I went to PC Richards, a electronics supply store, and purchased videocassettes on which I was going to record birthday messages for my young daughters to view in my absence.

Fortunately, the preliminary diagnosis was completely wrong. Dr. AO never apologized for the terror he caused for me for 5 days. After all, he said, "Why should I apologize? Would you have preferred if I was

THEY DIDN'T TEACH US THAT IN DENTAL SCHOOL

correct?" But for me, it was an epiphany. I vowed that I would never again miss a single one of my children's activities. I would go to every soccer game, tennis match, dance recital and orchestra performance because the opportunities to see your children develop, mature and achieve are limited. When you miss those events, they are lost forever. The opportunities to grow close with your spouse become threatened by many distractions if you do not devote sufficient time and energy to the relationship. By virtue of the decision I made as a result of my scare, I have no regrets for having always been "there" to cheer for my daughters athletic endeavors, to appreciate the development of musical and art talents, or to wipe the tears of joy and sadness from my wife's cheeks when things went either very well...or very bad. I was able to avoid getting caught up in "doing" by not losing sight of simply "being".

In the current environment there seems to be two strategies. Some are facing their adversity with complacency by waiting for conditions to improve. Others have concentrated their efforts on trying to implement multifaceted plans to counter challenging trends and have abandoned the sense of balance in their lives. Neither of these scenarios is positive in the long run.

Here are five techniques to bring a little more balance into your lives:

1. <u>Build downtime into your schedule</u>...make it a point to schedule time with family and friends

and activities that help you recharge. This will give you things to look forward to.

2. <u>Drop activities that sap your time and energy</u>...many people waste time on activities or people that add no value to your life. Minimize time spent with people who vent or gossip. Don't get sucked into habits that make you less efficient.

3. <u>Rethink tasks</u>...consider what responsibilities that you can delegate to others. Abandon the philosophy that "it won't get done right if I don't do it myself". Invest time in training others and communicating realistic expectations.

4. <u>Get moving</u>...find time for physical activity. Whether it's working out or playing a sport that you enjoy, there is a strong mind-body connection that enables you to achieve at a higher level in <u>all</u> of your endeavors.

5. <u>A little relaxation goes a long way</u>...even minor changes will start the process of regaining balance. Leave work an hour early one day each week or take an extra long weekend getaway during the course of the summer. During a hectic day, just take a 10 or 15-minute break to recharge your batteries.

Often times I will share with my family the ideas I'm considering for presentations and articles. When I shared the idea of "life balance" with my family over dinner one night I noticed two of my daughters rolling their eyes at each other. I prodded them to use their words and one of them said, "Dad, do you always practice what you preach?" This was probably said in response to the high number of presentations and articles I was writing as well as the work on this book. The reality check was good.

I need some practice with my own juggling skills. I need to insure that my glass balls stay afloat in the air and I maintain my sense of rhythm and balance. From time to time, I must also drop my rubber work ball to engage in more important pursuits. I, too, must drop my rubber work ball and maintain balance.

CHAPTER 29

Remembering Dr. Al Sternfeld

It is with a great deal of sadness that I am writing this remembrance of someone who was very dear to me. Dr. Alfred Sternfeld ("Al") was the gentleman that gave me my first opportunity in private practice nearly 30 years ago. Sadly, he passed away in January 2012 at the age of 97.

I was introduced to Al by an Oral Surgeon, who was an Attending from my residency, in the spring of 1984. We first met over lunch in his private office at his practice in Malverne, NY. There were turkey sandwiches cut in quarters on real plates. There was fruit "compote" in a glass parfait dish and a wine glass with club soda and 3 ice cubes. I remember this explicitly because every day that we had lunch together during the following two years, it was exactly the same. Al was an incredibly sweet and kind man with a reputation for being very difficult on the 20 associates that he had over the previous 25 years.

Rumors had it that he had fired two of his associates in the middle of procedures. (Remember this fact later on). He had a very clear vision of how perfect he wanted to run his practice and nothing distracted him from this goal.

We immediately hit it off and he quickly became my professional father, and I became his professional son. Though we had very different interests outside of dentistry, we were very connected within the office. Dr. Sternfeld's practice had a wonderful reputation and it was easy to see why.

He truly cared about his patients and they adored him with love and respect. He was one of the most skilled practitioners I had ever met and his work was exquisite and, as I have learned subsequently, certainly withstood the trials of time. He understood business, and even more so, people.

Our relationship inspired me from the very start. Four months after we met, Al gave me a vote of confidence and convinced me to take over the reins of his practice as he wanted to begin slowing down by just doing the dentistry he loved and not "running" the place. He was 70 at the time. The negotiations for this business transaction never occurred. There was little to contend. He was a generous and fair man. His handshake eliminated the need for attorneys, yet we both had our respective representatives. At the closing his attorney started to question some of our arrangements and Al fired him on the spot for interfering. My attorney completed the transaction. Dr. Sternfeld stuck by his word.

One of the conditions that Al insisted that we put in our contract was that for every day we would work together, we had to sit across the desk from each other and talk for 30 minutes over lunch, as described previously. How brilliant he was. I would have to describe something new clinically, whether it was a technique, a procedure, a material or a theory. He would have to tell me something about business, running the practice or dealing with people. I learned so much from him. I learned to respect how thirsty for knowledge he was. Even in the waning years of practice he wanted to learn and implement everything he could. It is partially because of Al that I have pursued over 4,000 hours of Continuing Education during my 30 years in practice. Most of all, I learned the importance of striving for perfection and committing to exceeding the expectations of those who we work with and for, our team and our patients.

As I travel around lecturing and consulting with fellow professionals in my role as a Coach and Consultant, much of what I teach I originally learned from Al. Al may have been soft spoken and diminutive in physical stature, but he was a giant in every other aspect of his presence.

Al taught me to become involved in my community. I followed him into the Rotary Club and eventually served a couple of terms as President. Al taught me to pursue interests away from the practice to create balance in my life. He was a ham radio enthusiast, a pilot, a captain of his sailboat, "Hey Ad" (Named after his wife of 56 years, Adelaide), and co-captain of the dinghy,

"Hey Al", which was always in tow with the "big boat" (The dinghy his wife named after him).

Few people know the real reason that Al retired in 1986. It is an event that fostered even more respect by me for him. Many years before that, he had once fired an associate for attempting a procedure that the young doctor was ill prepared to do because she felt that Dr. Sternfeld was "in the office in case she needed help". He said that it was bad judgment. One day early in 1986 Al came in to me to ask me for help with a difficult surgical extraction. Comfortable with the procedure, I thought nothing of it. Showing the utmost confidence in me, he left the room to allow me to complete what he had started. When I finished and had dismissed the patient I went to his office to tell him that everything had gone well. Surprisingly, I found that he had left the office and left me a note on the desk. The note said,

"Dear Steve, I have frequently told you how impor-tant it is to set your standards high and always abide by them. Today I showed bad judgment by attempting a procedure I had no business in performing." (Not really true). "For this I have chastised others. This lapse in judgment has convinced me that it is time to hang up my mirror and drill and pass the torch on to you. I leave you with much confidence that you will continue my legacy. Sincerely, Al"

I last spoke to Al in November, 2011. At the time he said he was struggling physically and mentally. His self-awareness was still remarkable. I reminded him of his note, but he did not recall leaving it for me. Well, I remember it every day. I still have the tooth that I completed extracting for him 25 years ago. To me it serves as a reminder to constantly strive for the highest standards in clinical performance, ethics and integrity. Al taught me as much about life as he did about dentistry. It is probably the reason why his patients loved him and continued to ask about him for 27 years with love and respect.

In my mind I see a horizon with a sailboat silhouetted by a sunset. With my binoculars all I can see are the words on the back of the dinghy being pulled by the bigger boat. "Hey, Al" we're gonna miss you.

Category Four: Sales

CHAPTER 30

Get Permission From <u>ALL</u> Of Your Patients To Provide Them With The Best Care Possible

O ne of the biggest mistakes that many dentists make is pre-judging the level of care desired by their patients. Face the fact that no person in his or her right mind will ever choose compromised care. People, in general, desire the highest quality of care possible, but they are often faced with obstacles unrelated to the care, itself, which may make the desired level of care seemingly unreachable. Our responsibility and that of our teams is, with outstanding verbal skills, to help our patients overcome these obstacles.

All too often there is a tendency to pre-qualify patients for treatment. "They won't be able to afford it," or "There's no way they will accept that much treatment" are the most common "excuses" for not presenting comprehensive care. These are more related to the dentist's state of mind than that of the patient. Many in our field are afflicted with "approval addiction". We are fearful that if a patient does not like, or approve, or is threatened by what we tell them, they will leave our practice and go elsewhere for care. If the messenger improves the delivery, the message will be received more openly.

My Coaching partner, Kelly Fox-Galvagni often tells the story of how she was humiliated when, as a single-mom/dental assistant, 20 years ago, she was told by an orthodontist that she wouldn't be able to afford treatment needed by her son, but he would develop an alternative course of treatment.

We suggest changing the relationship from the outset between the dentist and patient. Making patients feel that we are partners in their care, and not dictatorial, helps us create a much more receptive environment. One of the most valuable tools to achieve this is a dialogue called the "permission statement":

"Mrs. Jones, the doctor – patient relationship is extremely important to me. I would like your permission to be honest and truthful in everything I tell you concerning the condition of your mouth and how I would recommend caring for you…"

"The flip side of that is that I give you permission to ask any questions and make all decisions regarding your treatment. There are circumstances in your life that may impact on what treatment you do or not do and I trust and respect that. I want you to feel that we are partners in your care. How does that sound to you?"

The first part of the dialogue allows you to be thorough and honest without fear of rejection. The second part puts us in a position to help the patient overcome their challenges, whether they are monetary, psychological, time-related, trust-related or related to a perceived lack of urgency. There are verbal skills related to each of these challenges. The main point to understand here is that the decision to proceed with treatment is more related to a perceived level of value in the care than any other variable and our responsibility to the patient is to do everything possible to help build that perceived value. Understand the premise that as the perceived value goes up, the perceived cost goes down and this has more to do with the ultimate decision than any other factor. As you relate the dental treatment to emotional needs instead correcting clinical conditions your patients will absolutely place a higher level of importance and value in receiving your care.

CHAPTER 31

Focus On Value Over Price

Summer traveling has taken my wife and I to Starbucks in several different areas of the country. Wherever we have gone, my wife's coffees and my iced teas were identical. Similarly, if we were to purchase a can of Coke or a tube of Crest toothpaste anyplace in the country it will be exactly the same. This is what happens with commodities. Because they are the same it makes sense to differentiate based on price. The $2.49 tube of Crest in Costco is a smarter purchase than the $3.99 tube in your local boutique market. (Unless you place a "value" on the convenience of the local purchase.)

Dental insurance companies want dental care to become a commodity. If they can eliminate differentiation from the consideration of dental care, then they can also exert pressure to drive the "price" of dental care to a level prohibitively low for those providing the care. If our typical dental practices choose to "sell" dentistry based on price, then we are entering a losing battle in trying to compete with large dental corporations and emerging retail practices in stores like Wal-Mart with their overwhelming bulk-buying power.

We must promote dentistry as a "custom service" where value becomes the deciding factor. A commoditized practice has a set "price" for every procedure. A value-driven practice customizes solutions for each and every presenting condition based on the patient, the clinical presentation, the level of patient cooperation, the schedule and the level of expertise needed to solve the particular unique clinical situation.

Improving the quality of your service and customizing the aspects of your practice will increase the perceived value of your care. As the perceived value increases, the perceived cost decreases. Because patients will always invest in what they value, if they value their dental health and how you can contribute to it, then they will invest in your care. Always promote the benefits of your care and never lower the perceived value by competing on price.

CHAPTER 32

Why It's Important To Be Different

"Why is there always a cloud at the top of the mountain? Why do the sand crabs dig holes? Why do the birds dive into the water? Why can't we stay on vacation longer? Why are the dentists back home frustrated and unhappy? Why am I thinking about this on vacation?"

I still have no idea about the answers to the first three questions. I leave the answers to these questions to the meteorologists, the marine biologists and the ornithologists. The reason we couldn't stay longer is that I have three daughters, and someday I will have three weddings. The answer to the fourth question is because, as Bob Dylan said, "These times, they are changing." Like the dinosaurs, we are not adequately accommodating to the changes. The answer to the fifth question is because I truly care and my vision or belief is that I can make a difference in the lives of the people around me, in my practice, and in my profession.

What is your belief? What is your vision? Why do you practice dentistry? Why is it harder now? It is harder because as a profession we are not innovative. Sure, we adopt technology and we develop new techniques, but these are merely changes in what we do and how we do it. The challenge that we are facing is the commoditization of our profession. Insurance companies know it. Wal-Mart knows it. That is why these entities are so hell-bent on making "our" consumers think that our care is indistinguishable. A crown is a crown, isn't it? A filling is a filling, isn't it? A cleaning is a cleaning, isn't it? If all we are concerned with is what we do or how we do it, then the failure to differentiate will enable the proponents of commoditization to win.

Whenever we begin working with a practice we ask the doctor to tell us about their practice. *"I've had a successful practice." "We do quality work." "We have a gorgeous office." "We have the latest technology." "Every member of the team has 25 years of experience." "We do a lot of cosmetic dentistry." "We do implants." "We do Invisalign." "We have treated celebrities."*

If practicing dentistry were like dating, would this work at a party?

New Acquaintance: "So you're a dentist? What is that like?"

Dentist: "I've been very successful because I do quality work and have a beautiful office, the latest technology and a staff with each member having over 25 years of experience. I do a lot of cosmetic dentistry, implants and Invisalign and I have treated numerous celebrities. Would you like to make a "date" to come to my office?"

How do you think the dentist fared?

Unfortunately, many in our profession work very hard to prove their value without ever saying why they exist in the first place. They provide potential patients with a list of their experience, what they do and how they do it in the hope that the "prospects" will drop whatever they are doing and come to their practice. When you try to cultivate patients by defining what you do and how you do it, you are falling into the commoditization trap because it encourages those we serve into making their decisions based on intellect. They begin to weigh quality, service and cost like they do in clothing, groceries and appliances.

Now let's try the "dating" scenario with a different approach.

New Acquaintance: "So you're a dentist? What is that like?"

Dentist: "I love what I do. As a dentist, I love going to my office and working with an amazing group of experienced team members and wonderful patients whose lives we improve each and every day. Of course we have a beautiful office and the latest technology, but what excites me each and every day is that we make a difference in peoples' lives with cosmetic dentistry, implants and Invisalign. We've even had the opportunity to care for some celebrities and improve their lives, as well. May I invite you to come visit our wonderful office?"

Do you think this approach might have been more successful? Why? Exactly! People have less of an affinity for what we do than why we do it. People are inspired by beliefs, not by facts. When we have a greater sense of purpose in our practices we become less concerned with the aspects that may tend to make dentistry more of a commodity. This approach makes you different than most and patients are inspired by this difference.

When we promote dentistry by describing what we do or how we do it, a patient may think that coming to us is the right decision. That's what happens when we sift through the pros and cons of making a decision. Inevitably, there always remains some doubt because most people tend to second-guess the intellectual thought process. When a decision "feels" right we make "gut" decisions that seem to have a much greater level of confidence. We "trust our gut" because these decisions are usually based on congruence of beliefs. These beliefs are expressed to the patients when we emphasize why we do what we do instead of describing what we do or how we do it.

I understand that to differentiate you and your practice this way may seem like a difficult paradigm shift for the way most of you view dentistry. I also understand that this philosophy may need much greater clarification than can be achieved in this format.

For those of you who have detected some level of stagnation in your offices, you may be wondering why you should consider making such a drastic change in the way you differentiate your practices. My answer to those who feel this way is "WHY NOT?"

Mark Twain once said, *"The two most important days in your life are the day you were born and the day you found out why."*

CHAPTER 33

Objections Are Opportunities

"Back in the day" during the "Golden Age of Dentistry" a dentist was assured success merely by outfitting an office and hanging out a shingle. Dentists were overwhelmed with a deep schedule filled with patients wanting to "fix" their teeth with MODBL wraparound amalgams, "adaptic" composites and gold "veneer" crowns. Life was simpler for our patients. There was the early abundance of the "Baby Boom" era and seemingly little competition for the discretionary funds allotted to "fixing" one's teeth. There was little confusion with dental insurance as it could only help and the benefits allowed were reasonable for the fees that were charged.

A great deal has changed since that time. The "Baby Boom" generation has given rise to multiple industries, which seduce this population's desires to look good, feel well and have fun. Consumer electronics is a $1.3 trillion industry. The automobile industry shows revenues of $609 billion. Entertainment yields $500 billion and Fashion pulls in $300 billion. Dentistry, by comparison has become a smaller "player" at $110 billion. The difference is that years ago people "needed" dental treatment and they readily paid to have it done. Today, they want many expensive "things" more that the dentistry they need. Our industry has tried to help keep dentists in the forefront of things that people want with the development of cosmetic materials and procedures. The cosmetic results that we are able to achieve with smile design, ceramics and resins, and even whitening should have boosted our success in having patients choose dentistry over other indulgences. There has been a huge disconnect in dentists being able to overcome their view that dentistry is needed more than the truism that it is optional. In nearly every practice I visit, dentists and their teams exhaust themselves "educating" patients about what they need and they then become frustrated when patients say, "Doctor, I'll think about it." or "I'll do the fillings, but I'm going to wait on the crowns." We need to guide our patients into making better "emotional" decisions about their care.

The town of Brookhaven, NY failed to clear the roads following a blizzard in the winter of 2012-2013 when the Highway Superintendent, Michael Murphy, claimed to be paralyzed by the agony of a toothache. I feel the cause of this problem may have been a dentist who failed to make Mr. Murphy "want" to come for treatment of an existing problem before it became a debilitating condition.

Realize that our success is not dependent on educating our patients and telling them what they need to have done, but rather working in conjunction with our entire team to inspire our patients to want to care for situations in their mouth, which may have a greater impact on other aspects of their life. One of my most requested presentations is "A Team Approach to Successful Treatment Acceptance". This presentation is 100% geared to helping dentists and their teams master the skills to achieve improved case acceptance.

The alternative to patients dismissing their need for treatment and leaving with statements like I've listed previously, and having some interest, is when they begin to ask questions. From what we have seen, most dentists view the concept of questions as potential objections to treatment. Nothing could be further from the truth. The fact that a patient asks questions means that on some level, they have connected with the concept of treatment and they are looking for the doctor or treatment coordinator to help them through the intellectual concerns of their emotional "want".

The perceived objections to treatment usually surface with questions about 5 very distinct potential barriers.

1. Cost
2. Fear
3. Time
4. Need or sense of urgency
5. Trust

If you and your team are able to help the patient satisfy their concern for whichever one, or more, of these issues is raised, then you will turn this potential objection into an opportunity to provide them with the care that you know they need and now, they want.

CHAPTER 34

The ONLY Guaranteed Way
To Attract New Patients

Many Dental Practice Management Consultants are bright, business-trained individuals who have identified that dentists are a very needy population for their knowledge of business models and strategy. Similarly, there is an abundance of Marketing and Advertising professionals who readily recommend that dentists dabble in various strategies of branding with a logo and slogan, developing a web presence, participating in social-networking, a media presence (TV and Radio), spray-and-pray direct mail marketing and personalizing every toothbrush, floss dispenser and lip balm that leaves your office.

As I speak to Dentists and Office Managers the struggles of attracting new patients usually comes up in conversation. Most attribute the difficulties to the economy (ongoing for the past 5 years) and insurance limitations. Unfortunately, or fortunately, for that matter, many of the practices indicate that they are not proactively doing anything specifically to "market" new patients. They are relying on "hope" as a strategy. Hope is not a strategy!

The only sure-fired; absolute, unequivocal, guaranteed things that you can do are ... all that you do in your practice to create a world-class experience. The ONLY guaranteed method of generating new patient flow is to turn your patients into raving fans of your practice. (I highly recommend the book, "Raving Fans" by Ken Blanchard and Sheldon Bowles.) Patient satisfaction is never enough. (Another great book is *"Customer Satisfaction is Worthless, Customer Loyalty is Priceless: How to Make Them Love You, Keep You Coming Back, and Tell Everyone They Know"* by Jeffrey Gitomer). When people view a movie, eat at a restaurant, or experience treatment in your practice, there are generally 4 levels of satisfaction or approval that they can walk away with.

1. Lousy or poor - This is the worst. It will generate negative word-of-mouth and potentially, unfavorable on-line reviews. Do whatever you can to avoid this scenario.
2. Fair - No one ever talks about fair. Patients who have had a fair experience are one interaction with someone who has had a great experience somewhere else, from leaving your practice.
3. Good - Good used to be good enough. Dental consumers are better informed and more savvy than they used to be. They expect good care and a good experience. Anything less than good is unsatisfactory. A good reputation is NOT enough to make someone want to switch to your practice.

4. Great - Great inspires people to change their plans. If you hear a movie is great, you try to go this coming Saturday night. If you hear a restaurant is great, you try to get a reservation. If a dental practice is great, patients are more likely to brag to their friends and their friends become motivated and inspired new patients in your practice. Great is the minimum level you should try to attain.

To succeed in practice today, you have to deliver consistently great care and provide an even greater level of service. In other words, unless you have a unified, people-first, patient-oriented culture, it will be difficult to build your practice going forward. Any practice CAN achieve this. Understand that you cannot achieve this level of care and service by emphasizing the results that you want to achieve. This would be putting the cart before the horse. When you focus on the results, it is difficult to get your teams on board because they need to be convinced that it's the right way to go. A much more effective idea is to concentrate on building "your" people first and then they will copy your example and take care of your patients in the ways that you prefer. Get your team acting with passion, compassion and commitment and everything else will fall into place. With creative leadership and astute management, you will be able to create a self-perpetuating cycle where the culture you provide feeds the energy of your team and they, in turn will be inspired to provide a more energetic and compassionate level of care and service for your patients.

I am dedicated to helping practices develop this type of culture. Understand that every practice has a culture, which occurs either intentionally or by accident. It is the culture of your practice that ultimately determines how successful and fulfilled you and the members of your team will be.

CHAPTER 35

Multiplication

A t a time when it is difficult to attract new patients, what if we could give you simple, unique strategies to multiply your new patient flow. These techniques are simpler than taking your next needed dental instrument from a superbly trained 4-handed clinical assistant.

1. Understand that women make 85% of the decisions on appointments in your office for themselves and the members of their family. When a new patient, especially a woman, calls your office and you are able to "close" on the concept of making their initial appointment, simply add, *"It's great that we have been able to schedule you for your first visit to our office. Do you have any other members of your family that you would like to make appointments for while we are on the phone?"*
The goal in accepting appointments from prospective new patients is to achieve 100% success. This technique allows for the possibility of achieving a success rate greater than

100% for scheduling initial visits from initial phone calls.

2. The second technique takes place in the hygienist's treatment room. It is not uncommon for hygienists to give an adult patient a toothbrush at the end of their appointment. At this point, why not ask the patient (again, especially if it is a woman) if she would like a new toothbrush for any of the members of her family who are not patients in the practice. Then at the time of the handoff (transition of power) to the administrative team the hygienist should say, *"Lois, I have given Ms. Sunshine a toothbrush for her husband, Robert and her daughter, Michelle. Perhaps you might like to find out if she would like to include them in our family of patients and schedule an appointment for them."* Then the Administrative Team member, Lois, can review the practices "Care-to-Share" program or whatever the practice has to reward patients for the confidence of making a referral.

Both of these techniques need to be rehearsed and role-played to make them become comfortable for the team members involved. But, both techniques are guaranteed to help multiply the number of new patients seen in your practice. Start today and let me know how it works out for you and your practice.

CHAPTER 36

Use It Or Lose It

As Smile Potential has grown I have been able to see trends among the offices that I have worked with. Keeping the schedule filled with PRODUCTIVE appointments seems to be a common challenge. During the last quarter of the year it is imperative to help patients who have insurance coverage utilize every last available penny of their coverage before it is lost. The first step is to send out a "Use It Or Lose It" letter to every patient who has insurance coverage in late September or early October. You may send these letters out by mail or email, if you have your patients' email addresses. Here is that letter:

"Dear Patient,
You would never think of taking your hard-earned money and tossing it out the window, but that's exactly what you'd be doing if you didn't make full use of your dental insurance benefits. Most dental insurance is based on a calendar year and if the dollar amount of coverage is not used, you lose those benefits. You could be throwing away several hundred to several thousand dollars in benefits that were either paid by

you directly or through salary deductions. With the rising cost of insurance, you may not have comparable benefits in the future. In addition, the New Year will begin with a new deductible that will have to be met by you.

The year is rapidly coming to an end. The enclosed page shows unfinished treatment that we have recommended to you for your well-being. You may have coverage remaining that could be used to help you pay for this care that you had indicated you wanted. Note that our estimated insurance figures may not be an accurate record of your insurance coverage. We recommend that you phone your carrier to find out definitively what coverage you have left.

Although our recommended treatment is never dictated by insurance policy limitations, our experience has shown that benefits can often be maximized through careful planning. We can often plan necessary care to take full advantage of your insurance coverage. We do not want you to be among those who lose valuable dental benefits. Call us now to make an appointment to begin or complete your treatment before the end of the year.

Sincerely,
Office Manager"

We recommend that in addition to this you go through your list of patients and determine who has benefits available at the end of September. For those who have unscheduled treatment or incomplete treatment plans, this is an opportunity to match up their available coverage with work that they want are aware of needing. For patients without treatment plans and significant coverage left, we encourage you to bring these patients in for a complimentary screening, for their benefit, to see if there is any work that can be done before the end of the year before they lose their benefits. In any case, we highly recommend phone calls to follow up any correspondence sent out by mail or email.

CHAPTER 37

Sustained Release Marketing

O ne of the most common marketing initiatives is to promote a "special" offering, whether it is a discounted service or a new service provided by the practice. It is not uncommon for offices to send out a huge mailing to their patients to prompt them to take advantage of whatever they are offering du jour, whether it is whitening, cosmetics, Invisalign, painless root canals, or something hygiene-related. The frustration comes when the response is poor and the effort seems to be a time-consuming, money-wasting endeavor. Often times the promotion is extremely worthwhile. The problem usually does not lie with the promotion, but rather in the method chosen to announce it.

I have found, and I recommend to our clients, to accumulate email addresses for all of your patients. Email is beginning to infiltrate even the most unlikely members of our patient population. At the very least, email is a terrific way to reach the vast majority of your patients today. It costs nothing and can be repeated as often as you want if you feel that the first attempt fell on blind eyes (I wanted something comparable to "deaf ears"). The problem with mass mailings and even mass e-mailings is the level of enthusiasm of the people receiving it. Even the most beautifully constructed email will soon leave the consciousness of the recipients. Do you ever notice how for the week or two following a mailing, some patients ask about it and then the interest starts to disappear?

What I recommend is to sustain the release of promotional marketing to take advantage of the phenomenon previously described. What we have found to work extremely well is to mail, whatever we would have mailed to everyone, to only the patients due in hygiene for the following week. We usually send it out on Tuesday or Wednesday so that they receive it before the weekend, when they are more likely to open it or read it. When they come in the following week, if they do not ask about the promotion, the hygienist enthusiastically asks if they received our letter or post card with the "great news". It gives us an opportunity to verbally reinforce the BENEFIT of what we are offering. Remember, we never promote treatment of any kind. We only promote the benefits of the treatment we are hoping to perform, whether it is enhanced appearance, looking younger, relieving discomfort, improving function, improving their love life or losing weight. (OK, the last two are wishful thinking that we may not be able to help with.) We are not concerned if patients receive more than one card because of repeated hygiene visits for soft-tissue management or quarterly periodontal maintenance. If we notice it, by chance, we can eliminate a repeat mailing. More important is the fact that over a period of 6 months every patient on recall for twice per year will receive this promotion.

The bottom line is that I have found this program is highly effective in getting the word out about our promotions and we have noticed a significantly higher interest in our patients in taking advantage of what we are offering. This has contributed to our increased production and profitability.

SECTION THREE:

The 15 Most Frequently Asked Questions And Other Scripts

Excellent verbal skills are essential for creating exceptional customer service. The use of effective scripts can help a dental team enhance their verbal skills. Scripting is the single most important team-training tool in the development of excellent verbal skills.

In my presentations to Dentists and team members, I speak extensively about the development of comprehensive job descriptions and practice procedure manuals. The systems that result from this type of documented organization are what create efficiency in any practice, big or small. **Systems run the practice and people run the systems.** In too many offices that I have visited, nearly all of the important information is held in the "heads" of the team members. The Administrative team member knows what is going on in patients personal lives, when they are available to schedule, personal situations that are preventing them form scheduling, how they pay for treatment, who referred them and who they have referred. Rarely is this information organized in a manner that other team members could access the information. When it is

169

recorded it is usually indecipherable in a wire-bound note-book.

The hygienist knows patient treatment preferences, where they have sensitive areas, what motivates them for treatment, what demotivates them for treatment and what the doctor told them "last time" they were in. Our dental assistants know where everything we use is located. They keep track of inventory in their heads. They know and anticipate what we need, often times before we know it. Unfortunately, the "hard drives" of their knowledge are not transplantable to their successors.

The example that I like to use describes a dental team of three, similar to those I have described above, who together purchase a Power Ball or Mega Millions ticket for $150 million on Friday afternoon. What happens when their numbers win the grand prize during the course of that weekend? With $150 million divided among them, how many of them do you think return to work on Monday morning raring to go for a full day of caring for patients? The only reason they show up on Monday is to collect their things and say goodbye. With their departure, all of the knowledge that they have been storing in their heads leaves with them. Where does that leave the doctor? "Up a creek without a paddle" doesn't come close to describing the inconvenience of trying to recover and recreate the lost knowledge that left with the team.

In 2009 I experienced, first hand, the benefits of having well-defined systems in my practice. Beginning in March of that year, one-by-one, five members of my team came to me to inform me that they were pregnant and due to deliver in the month of September. Included in this group were two of my three administrative team members, a full-time hygienist and two of my dental assistants. In addition, my third administrative team member was leaving in September to return to school. Fortunately, my office manager, Mercedes, who was one of the "expecting", had developed and organized a practice operations manual of close to 1,000 pages that described, in detail, every function of every position in the practice. This included where switches were located and how to turn equipment on and off, photos of setups and how each instrument was used, screen shots of all computer functions and flow charts for computer processes. There wasn't a single process or procedure that was not described. The result is that during the final quarter of that year we were able to generate the best numbers in the history of the practice...with six new or temporary team members.

Scripting is a direct extension of the systems development for a practice. When team members are able to present a unified, clear and consistent message to patients it builds confidence. One of the worst scenarios is for a patient to ask the same question of different members of the team and to get an equal number of different answers. As an experiment take aside each member of your own teams and independently ask them the following questions. When you have finished, review and compare their answers. What would a patient have thought from the assortment of responses?

- What is a root canal?
- Why can't I just have a filling?
- What do I need to do after I have an extraction?
- How long will my veneers last?

- When should I bring my child to her first dental visit?
- Can I make payments for my treatment?
- What is the doctor's background and experience?
- Should a specialist do this procedure?

What you will find from this exercise is that in many cases some of our team members have no idea of what to say. They may respond to these questions with things that they've heard in prior offices. They may be guessing because they fear that they have to say something. If they shy away from answering it may evoke hesitance in a patient.

Scripted positive language creates enthusiasm and motivation for treatment because it builds value for the practice's services. Most important, it guides conversation to emphasize patient benefits.

As with almost any training, if scripting is not practiced regularly, it will fall by the wayside. Scripts need to become a habit. Each member of the team on a regular basis must review the "Script Book" for a practice, at least once a month. I also suggest periodic role-playing to practice the scripts in simulated situations. The other purpose of role-playing is to enable team members to individualize or personalize scripts to their level of comfort, while still offering the same information.

The following list of questions and responses should be a key part of any practices "Script Book". One of the first exercises I give any practice which has engaged Smile Potential in a Coaching capacity is to make a list of the 25 most common questions asked of members of the team during he course of an average day, week or month. Every practice is different and each practice has different questions. Once this list is formulated, then I work with the team in developing concise, benefit-oriented scripts of responses that would reflect the practice in the most positive light. The responses listed on the following pages are examples of he types of responses that I recommend for the 15 most common questions. I suggest that they be used as a basis to develop your own responses to similar questions. I would be happy to review any responses that you and your teams develop. Contact me at the email address: SmilePotential@aol.com.

QUESTION 1:

Do you take my insurance?

This is far and away the most common question that practices say is number one on their lists. Understand that patients calling a new practice for the first time are generally nervous...and ignorant. They simply do not know what to ask. It has taken, for many, a degree of courage to make the call in the first place and the level of commitment can be variable. Many of the prospective patients asking this question actually got your name off their insurance company's website, yet they still ask. Also understand that the best response to many questions is another question. The reason for this is that it helps you determine what they were "really" asking in the first place.

With this being said, we recommend responding to this question with the counter question:

"How did you hear about our office?"

If the patient relates that they got your name off their insurance company's website, then it is an easy, affirmative slam-dunk.

If the patient says that they were referred by "Suzy Sunshine", one of your very best patients, who has had extensive treatment and has referred others, then you

have some leverage in knowing that insurance participation may not be a limiting factor due to influenced
trust.

If the patient has not indicated what coverage they
have, there is no reason to definitively declare whether
or not you are a participant in their plan:

*"We are an insurance-friendly practice and find
that we work successfully with all insurance plans.
Why don't you bring your benefits book with you to
your first appointment and we can do a complimentary benefits check for you?"*

This is where I usually get the reaction that we are
not being honest or that I am misleading patients. This
is emphatically not the case. On an initial visit most
plans will pay a significant portion of your diagnostic
fees. If they do not, I am willing to "gift" the occasional
disappointment to let a prospective new patient see the
type of practice that we are. Many have then committed
to extensive treatment independent of their coverage.
As a side note, many individuals who have lousy insurance are financially able to sustain significant care and
are not "prisoners" to lousy insurance coverage that was
contracted by the HR department of their employer.

If a patient relates an insurance company that you
do not participate in, respond with an answer that
engages every person's need to feel that they "belong"
in a particular situation:

*"We have had many patients in our practice who
have had your same insurance coverage. Many of*

them have had extensive treatment and have appreciated how we have maximized their coverage."

Understand that the "only" purpose of a "New Patient" phone call is to get the prospective patient in the door. Once they arrive, with an amazing first experience, you have the opportunity to convince them that it is in their best interest to make decisions independent of their insurance coverage. If you practice with this mindset, you will be surprised at how many patients will place a greater priority on the quality of their care than their level of reimbursement. As we develop this type of independence in our practices, the scope of our dentistry expands and our profitability increases.

QUESTION 2:

Do I really need a crown?

This is a perfect example about the type of question that sounds direct, but is really quite vague. It is the type of question that certainly demands greater clarification to determine what is the motive for the question. Does it pertain to trust or cost, which seem to be the likely reasons for the question. Or is it an indirect way to ask about fear, time or sense of urgency. For this reason, this question would best be clarified by asking another question?

"Mrs. Jones, does your concern about the need for a crown stem from fear of the procedure or some other reason?"

Once the patient is given the opportunity to clarify the question, it enables us to use some of the strategies that will be outlined for the following questions.

QUESTIONS 3:

Why does it cost so much?

P atients need to be reminded that quality care is an investment in their health and their potential level for success, both socially and professionally. It is important to bring them back to conversations that you have had with them about their chief complaints, or conditions that they presented with. Then we need to reconnect the conversation to the "disabilities" that were associated with the conditions, embarrassment, self-consciousness, self-confidence (for cosmetic conditions), distraction, frustration, inability to focus (for complaints of pain), difficulty chewing, annoyance, quality of life (for missing teeth or ill-fitting prosthetics). Focusing on these "disabilities" increases the perceived value of the care (which should be geared towards the disability) and when you raise the perceived value, you also decrease the perceived cost, making it more likely that the patient will choose to proceed with treatment.

When discussing prospective treatment, even before diagnosis has occurred, it is useful to engage patients in the conversation of anticipated investment. At the point where a patient has acknowledged that they have many "needs" and may want a solution that you can provide, it may be useful to ask the patient:

"Have you considered a budget for your dental care?"

This question will give you an idea of the patient's reality base and also some insight into their previous history. It may indicate the need to educate the patient before overwhelming them with proposed treatment.

Understand that there are 5 main objections to treatment: cost, fear, time, sense of urgency and trust. It is also important to realize that the expression of any of these objections indicates interest on some level of proceeding with treatment and, therefore, these objections should be considered your opportunities to proceed with care, once the objections are solved. The patient is looking to you to help them resolve these conflicts.

The best first response to the question of cost is:

"Is it the total cost of your treatment, or if we could fit the investment into a workable cash flow or budget, would it enable you to proceed with treatment?"

If the patient has been sufficiently motivated to pursue treatment, this is an enabling offer to help them overcome the objection of cost. Once the patient embraces the idea of budgeting it opens up the possibility to offering the concept of "payments over time with no interest". Notice I did not say to offer a third party financing plan, but to instead offer the budgeting solution. Only after the concept is accepted do you then offer the third party financing option. In this circumstance, I believe the best company to deal with is CareCredit.

QUESTION 4:

What is a crown (inlay, onlay)?

When answering questions about clinical treatments it is important to remember that the patient has very little connection to the clinical treatments for conditions that they may present with. With that being said, it is important to redirect the question to enable it to be responded to with a discussion of benefits and resolution of disabilities caused by conditions in the mouth. Begin the response to this question with a reminder to the patient of the "problem" that they own. Then immediately follow this with benefits of treatment.

"Mrs. Jones, if you recall from the photograph that I had on the monitor, you have a tooth that is decayed, fractured and the filling in that tooth has failed. If we left this tooth the way it is it will cause pain, it may fracture and it may need to be removed. In order to get rid of the decay, prevent it from hurting, replace the lost tooth structure, strengthen the tooth, make it last longer and look beautiful I have recommended the best way of treating that tooth, which is to restore it with a crown (or inlay or onlay). Do you have any questions?"

QUESTION 5:

Can the treatment wait?

This may also be a question about fear or cost, but more likely it is a question concerning "sense of urgency". It is important to always validate a patients concern, relate it to a similar concern that other patients have had and then tap into the inner need to derive security from "following the pack". This is called the "feel, felt, found" closing.

"Mrs. Jones, I know exactly how you feel. Other patients have felt exactly the same way, but they have found that by following the doctor's recommendation they were able to avoid the problems of pain and possible loss of he tooth. In light of this, doesn't it make good sense to proceed with the treatment?"

QUESTION 6:

Will I have pain?

This question is clearly derived from fear. It is important to be reminded of the fact that none of us were born with dental fear. Dental fear is either derived from a bad experience on the part of the patient, or it is implied through interactions with friends, family and co-workers.

"Mrs. Jones, that is certainly a valid concern. Have you previously had a bad experience?"

At this point the patient will usually describe either a bad previous experience or relay a horror story passed on to them from a friend or acquaintance. This is the point where you can begin differentiate yourself from the "other guy" and build up that differentiation into an advantage.

"I am sorry that you had that experience (or that you heard about that experience). However, I want to assure you that Dr. Wonderful is very empathic to your concern for discomfort and he/she is willing to do everything and anything necessary to insure that you are comfortable. Does that give you some sense of comfort in moving ahead in your treatment? If you feel anything that is uncomfortable just give the doctor a little hand signal and he/she

will stop immediately to give you more medication to make you comfortable."

The last part of this statement is designed to give the patient a feeling of control. Loss of control is often times more fear provoking than the concern for pain. It is very comforting to the patient to know that they have the ability to control their environment.

QUESTION 7:

How long will the veneers last?

The question about how long treatment will be successful is clearly a question about value. It implies an assumption that the treatment has been accepted and now the "value-added" feature is that, either the patient will "get their money's worth", or that they will not have to experience this process again anytime soon. Since the question is about value, this answer should clearly review the benefits and introduce some "cheerleading".

"Remember how badly chipped (or fractured, or decayed) this tooth was before we started? The treatment that Dr. Wonderful performed will not only fix what was unhealthy (or unsightly) but it will strengthen the tooth and enable you to enjoy it for a long time. This is because Dr. Wonderful uses the latest techniques, the best materials and he has constantly attended continuing education to insure that your veneers will last as long as possible."

Sometimes an elderly patient will make reference to their age in the discussion of whether they should proceed with treatment. Many years ago, Mr. Brown, a 97 year-old patient, presented to my office with his great-granddaughter accompanying him. Mr. Brown wanted nice new "caps" on his front teeth so that he could smile at his new girlfriend in the nearby assisted living facility. Mr. Brown had robbed the cradle with this relationship. His girlfriend was 86. The day that we cemented his porcelain crowns Mr. Brown looked in the mirror and asked, *"Hey Katz, how long are these things going to last me?"* My assistant looked at me and giggled and I turned to Mr. Brown and confidently stated, *"Mr. Brown, I'm going to give you my lifetime guaranty."* This was a very safe promise in consideration of his age. Mr. Brown quickly shot back, *"Katz, I don't need any of this lifetime crap. All I need is 10 years out of them because I don't think she's going to last any longer than that."* God bless Mr. Brown. He made it to 103...and the veneers did outlast his girlfriend, who had passed away a few months before he did.

My favorite statement when this topic comes up is:

"Mrs. Jones, this is where you and I have very different goals. My goal is to provide you with care that will last you a lifetime. Your goal is to outlive it."

I'm convinced that Mr. Brown smiles down on me whenever I say this line.

QUESTION 8:

Is there an alternative treatment?

This question is usually about cost, though fear and time may enter into the equation. Therefore it is again important to ask a qualifying question so that there can be clarity in your response.

"Mrs. Jones, is the reason for your question because it pertains to cost, or is it something else?"

Assuming it is cost, you must then, either return to the script for question number 3, "Why does it cost so much?" or, in the interest of seeing your patient through to the point of receiving treatment, you might begin a conversation of "phasing" treatment over an extended period of time. The advantage of this is that the patient is still able to receive the recommended care at a pace that is affordable for them.

"Mrs. Jones, a few moments ago you were quite clear in your desire to have the type of care that I recommended to you. Unless you are in a hurry, does it make sense to continue with this plan and just take our time to enable you to keep up with the finances and not feel over-burdened? I would be happy to make the arrangements to extend this treatment over a longer period of time, which will enable you to utilize more of your insurance benefits and still receive the care that you wanted."

QUESTION 9:

Is this a common procedure?

Remember that a high percentage of the patients we treat fall into the personality type of being introverted and people-oriented. Those that fall into this set of traits have a strong need to feel that they are part of a group, that they have things in common with others and that they are not alone. Most people do not want to "stand out", even if it is just in their own mind.

More importantly, though this is a "trust" question, a patient's confidence is higher if they feel that the care that they are receiving is "routine".

"The predictability and success of treatment is directly proportional to the level of skill and experience of the doctor. Because Dr. Wonderful has received so much additional continuing education and he/she has performed your procedure so many times during his/her career, in his/her hands this is a relatively common procedure."

QUESTION 10:

Why don't I feel it?

Patients are generally under the misconception that unless they feel something, everything is fine. In spite of the fact that we have been taught about the "silent" killers in medicine, dentistry has never been able to fully occupy this level of awareness.

My suggested response to questions about a void in perceived symptoms is relatively facetious, but it is effective in convincing the patient that preventive care is often times the smarter way of engaging treatment.

"Mrs. Jones, with regard to your question about the teeth not hurting...YET, here is my advice...If you would prefer not to begin treatment now, I want you to promise me that you will absolutely call me to begin treatment the day before it breaks, fractures, or starts causing you excruciating pain."

When this statement is used, patients will frequently call the practice back soon after they have left the office to schedule an appointment.

QUESTION 11:

At what age should I bring my child?

O bnoxiously, I am not going to answer this question because the answer, for the purposes of this book, is unimportant. There is no other question that does a better job of demonstrating the importance of scripted answers than this one. The most important thing to remember is that consistency in the message, throughout the team, breeds confidence. If the administrative team member answers this question by saying "3 years", the doctor says "2 years" and the hygienist says "18 months" it is confusing, at best, to a new mother. Confusion translates into lowered confidence. It is for this reason that I recommend that the practice team discuss this question at a Team Meeting and adopt it as the policy of the practice. It should periodically be reviewed to determine if the standard survives the test of time.

QUESTION 12:

Can I skip the x-rays?

The reluctance to have x-rays taken usually falls under two main objections. The first objection stems form the fear of effects of radiation. In the litigious society that we live in, physicians, mainly, have been forced to perform far more tests than are absolutely necessary to cover their derrieres. Individuals who have been pursuing any medical treatment have usually been bombarded with a battery of tests and x-rays. Certainly, one of the technologies that enable one to confidently answer this question affirmatively is the utilization of digital radiography.

"Mrs. Jones, Dr. Wonderful shares your concern about safety of radiology. It is for this reason, that he invested in technology to reduce your radiation exposure by over 90%. This reduces your exposure to radiation to less than watching TV or sitting in the sun."

The second reason some patients may choose to refuse x-rays is that they think that if they avoid the x-rays, it will limit our ability to give them "bad" news. The fact of the matter is that by avoiding x-rays, often times situations go undetected until they become symptomatic, indicative of more difficult and costly care.

"Mrs. Jones, I hear your reluctance to have any x-rays taken at this time. In order to make an accurate diagnosis, your physician will take your blood pressure, draw "bloods" and perform an EKG. In order to make an accurate diagnosis and to determine that everything is OK in your mouth, it is necessary for us to take x-rays. Won't you please reconsider?"

The gist of this response is that no one I know would ever want an "inaccurate" diagnosis.

QUESTION 13:

What are your hours?

Over the last few years we have been led to believe that unemployment has been a major challenge to our practices. Even at 10% unemployment, that means 90% of our patients have still been gainfully employed. The fallout of the economic climate is that everyone is being forced to work harder and longer to derive the same benefit. This means that patients who used to be able to take off time from work for a dental appointment are no longer able to do so. To this end, I recommend making early morning, and I mean very early morning, appointments available for some of your patients so that they may have treatment rendered even before they board their normal trains and buses for work.

This is a statement that I use routinely in describing our willingness to expand our hours, *"Mr. Jones, we find it is often helpful to make our schedule flexible because your schedule may not be."*

QUESTION 14:

Can you just bill me?

One of the best measures of the health of a practice is tracking the percentage of payments that are received "over the counter" at the time of service. I find that the practices with the healthiest cash flows are usually hovering around 70-75% of payments at the time of service. In most practices this takes a tremendous amount of re-training of the patients to comply with this sort of policy. Inevitably, there is pushback to keep the status quo of "take my insurance and bill me for the balance." Remembering to always present a benefit before you present treatment, the same holds true when presenting a policy.

"Mrs. Jones, our patients seem to appreciate everything that we do to keep our care affordable. One of the things that we have decided to do to help us keep your cost down is to reduce the amount of time and expense that we devote to billing. In order to keep your fees down we ask that you pay for your portion of the bill today, at the time of treatment. In order to further save you some money, I can save you 5% on todays bill if you will make the payment in full at this time. Doesn't it make sense to take advantage of this savings?"

QUESTION 15:

Is the doctor running on time?
(See Chapter 9: SOOT-SOT-GOOT)

As was mentioned earlier, failure to respect the time of others is, perhaps, the most damaging practice that you can engage in. Conversely, being respectful of others time can be a major practice builder. Through the use of procedure time studies and conscientious scheduling it is important to allow adequate time for all procedures. This precludes trying to "squeeze" extra procedures into an inadequate amount of time. It is terribly counter productive. Even in the most carefully constructed schedule, however, the nature of our business is that an emergency or an unforeseen event during a procedure can throw a wrench into our punctuality. When this occurs it is important to still be respectful of the time of your subsequent patients. When possible, it is preferred to try to call these patients before they leave to come to our offices. If this was not possible, however, it is important to convert the negative into a positive by dealing with the situation in the most positive way possible. What I recommend is for the doctor to come out to the reception room and speak to the subsequent patient. Leaving your surgical cap and loupes on during this conversation lends even more credibility to the gesture.

"Mrs. Jones, despite my constant effort to run on time, occasionally things come up in the form of emergencies, which cause me to disappoint my wonderful patients, like yourself. I apologize that I am running behind and I will not be able to see you for another 15 (20, 30, 45 minutes). If this will be inconvenient for you I completely understand if you would like to reschedule now for a new appointment. If it is not inconvenient I will be happy to see you as soon as I am finished with this appointment and know that I will absolutely devote the originally intended amount of time to your procedure as well."

Regardless of the patients decision, add, *"For your inconvenience, I would like to offer you a gift card to either Dunkin Donuts or Starbucks, whichever you prefer. I respect your schedule and I apologize for making you wait."*

Patient Interview Questions

Strengths:
- *"What are some good experiences that you had in your last dental office?"*
- *"What are you looking for in a dental practice?"*
- *"What makes you feel comfortable in a dental office?"*

Weaknesses
- *"Sounds like you had a bad experience. Would you please share it with me?"*
- *"What do you dislike about going to the dentist?"*
- *"What are some fears that you have about going to the dentist?"*

Opportunities:
- *"If you could change anything about your teeth, what would it be?"*
- *"Some people are interested in function. Some in looks. What is important to you?"*
- *"If there were nothing standing in your way, what would you like for your teeth?"*

Threats:

- *"Would there be any reason not to get needed dental treatment done?"*
- *"Is there any reason you could or would not get your dental work taken care of?"*
- *"If your insurance company doesn't pay for a procedure, what steps would you like to take to handle those?"*

Office Tour

- *"In order to make you feel at home..."*
- Everything is presented with benefit statements:
- Common areas: *"In order to make you as comfortable as possible..."*
- Treatment rooms: *"In order to provide you with the best care possible..."*
- Sterilization: *"In order to insure your safety, our office exceeds all requirements for sterilization and cleanliness..."*
- Bathroom: *" For your comfort we have a nice selection of toiletries for you to freshen-up"*

Permission Statement

(See Chapter 26)

"Mrs. Jones, the doctor – patient relationship is extremely important to me. I would like your permission to be honest and truthful in everything I tell you concerning the condition of your mouth and how I would recommend caring for you..."

"The flip side of that is that I give you permission to ask any questions and make all decisions regarding your treatment. There are circumstances in your life that may impact on what treatment you do or not do and I trust and respect that. How does that sound to you?"

Retracted Smile Photo

- *"Mrs. Jones, I just put up on the computer monitor the picture that we took earlier in the appointment of your smile. Please tell me what your impression is of your smile. What is it that you like about it?"*
- If patient says they <u>love</u> their smile: *"That's wonderful. So few of our patients feel that way. Dr. Wonderful has developed an outstanding reputation and is extremely well respected for doing <u>exquisite</u> cosmetic dentistry and smile enhancement. Many of our patients have chosen to have the doctor develop a plan for improving their smiles. If you know of anyone who could benefit from this type of care please let me or any my team know and we can reach out to them for you."*
- If patient <u>does not</u> indicate that they <u>love</u> their smile: *"Dr. Wonderful has developed an outstanding reputation and is extremely well-respected for doing <u>exquisite</u> cosmetic dentistry and smile enhancement. If you had the opportunity, is there anything about your smile that you would like to change?"*
- *"May I share with Dr. Wonderful what we just spoke about?"*

- When Dr. comes in: *"I just had the opportunity to discuss with Mrs. Jones her thoughts about her smile. This is what she shared with me……….. Is there anything that you might recommend to address her concerns?"*

Triple Hear

O ne of the best ways to gain acceptance of proposed treatment is to engage in repetition in the message to the patient regarding their ownership of a problem, co-diagnosis of the importance to correct that problem and acceptance of the recommended treatment. To accomplish this at the highest level requires rehearsed, coordinated and choreographed interaction between the hygienist and patient, hygienist and doctor, doctor and patient, hygienist and treatment coordinator and treatment coordinator and patient. Each time the patient hears the message it further reinforces the message of importance on all levels mentioned previously.

The conversations go like this:

Hygienist to patient, *"Mrs. Jones, as you can see on this picture of the tooth on the upper right, there is decay, a fracture and a broken filling. If left untreated, this will cause you pain and may even cause you to lose this tooth. In order to fix what is broken, prevent you from having pain or getting an infection, to restore the tooth, strengthen it, make it last longer and look like a beautiful new tooth, Dr. Wonderful will probably recommend that you have a crown made."*

Then when the doctor enters the hygiene room for a "check", *"Dr. Wonderful, as you can see on the screen, there is a tooth with decay, a fracture and a broken filling. I've explained to Mrs. Jones that if left untreated, this will cause her to have pain and may even cause her to lose this tooth. In order to fix what is broken, prevent her from having pain or getting an infection, to restore the tooth, strengthen it, make it last longer and look like a beautiful new tooth, I've explained that you will probably recommend that she have a crown made."*

After the doctor examines the tooth, *"Mrs. Jones, Francine has correctly identified a tooth with decay, a fracture and a broken filling. If left untreated, this will cause you to have pain and may even cause you to lose this tooth. In order to fix what is broken, prevent you from having pain or getting an infection, to restore the tooth, strengthen it, make it last longer and make it look like a beautiful new tooth, I am going to recommend that you have a crown made."*

Shade Measurement

- *"Mrs. Jones, I am just going to take a measurement of the shade of your front teeth for our record."*
- (Take out light-to-dark shade guide): *"This guide shows the range of shades of most people's teeth ranging from light-to-dark. This is where your teeth fall on this range."* (Point to corresponding tab) *"Are you aware that whitening your teeth could result in your shade being lightened to somewhere in this range?"* (Point to shade tabs 6-8 spots over from the patient's). *"Is that something that might interest you?"*
- If yes...you should know what to do.
- If no... *"Well, this may not be something that interests you now, but if at any time in the future you might want to whiten your teeth for a special event, please let me know."*

Intraoral Photography / Quadrant Dentistry

"As you can see in the photo your old metal fillings are failing. They are cracked and grossly decayed. Since decay seems to travel from tooth to tooth, if we treat the worst one first and leave the others, the decay may return to the tooth we worked on. Doesn't make sense to take care of all three of these teeth at this time?"

Appointment Cancellation

1. Sound surprised and say, *"Oh!"*
2. *"Please hold while I pull your chart"*
3. Review importance of appointment and ask, *"Is there any possible way to keep this appointment which was reserved for you?"*
4. If productive appointment, ask to "hold" again while you try to put the Doctor on the line.
5. Patient will frequently change mind, rather than disturb the doctor or doctor may be able to regain commitment.

Patient Satisfaction Calls

- The Doctor should make daily post-op phone calls to any patient who receives anesthetic. *"I just wanted to make sure that you were doing OK. Do you have any questions?"*
- Patient satisfaction calls should be made by the Patient Coordinator 1-2 weeks after treatment is completed. *"Dr. Wonderful just wanted to make sure that you were 100% satisfied with your treatment. Do you have any questions?"*
- If there has been any problem, this is an opportunity to get the patient back in to correct the problem or "perceived problem."
- If the patient indicates they are completely satisfied, **this is an opportunity to ask for a referral.**

Asking For Referrals

- <u>Does not</u> imply desperation
- <u>Does</u> imply PRIDE

"Mrs. Jones, would it be possible for you to do a favor for me? You've mentioned that you are happy with the result of your treatment. We are also proud of what we've accomplished together. Could you please think of the names of one or two people who you think could benefit from our level of care. We would welcome your friends and family as guests in our practice."

Section Four:

I Appreciate You's

The first person who I want to thank is my incredible wife, Regina. She has supported me ever since we were undergraduate students together at Columbia University, where we met in September 1975. After marriage, she supported me, financially as well as emotionally, while I was in Dental School and while she was pursuing her Masters degree at the School of Social Work, at Washington University. I thank her for her tolerance of my schedule and for helping me to control my excitement and exuberance when ideas strike me at all hours of the day and night.

Next I want to express appreciation to my daughters, Heather, Nicole and Allison for always "Keeping Me Real" (see Chapter 22). They all know that much of my speaking has incorporated the areas of motivation and staying positive. Leave it to my daughters to "burst my bubble" when I've either lost my temper or exhibited frustration over something around the house, when they confront me with *"Way to go Mr. Positive Thinking. What would your clients or audiences say if they could see you now?"*

Much of what I talk about in Coaching, Lectures and in this book is derived from my Dental Practice, Smiles On Broadway, in Malverne, Long Island. Most of what we do has been perfected with the input of my wonderful team. Within my practice I want to acknowledge three team members in particular. Denise has been a superb assistant in the practice for over 15 years. I always appreciate her professionalism, her work ethic and her dedication to travel over an hour each way in her 80-mile round-trip commute to the office. Francine has been the primary hygienist in my practice, also for 15 years. Francine is the most compassionate person I have ever worked with and in recent years, she has also proven to be the most courageous. Mercedes was the office manager of my practice during the re-emergent years of double-digit growth. She was a strong leader who embraced systems and progress. I miss her.

Kelly Fox-Galvagni has been my partner in Smile Potential Dental Practice Coaching since we began in 2009. When it comes to Dental Practice Management, our minds function as one. We think alike and know what the other one is going to say before they do. It is a pleasure to work with her.

I want to also thank my buddies from my DDS "support group". Drs. Steve Boral, Fred Danziger, Bob Berg, Barry Goodman, Jay Piskin and I have been meeting on Monday evenings for 28 years. During this time we have counseled and supported each other in practice-related and personal challenges. It is an intimate group built on deep trust and sincere caring. Thank you for always being there when I've needed you guys.

I want to thank my friend, Mark Marinbach, from Nu-Life Long Island Dental Lab, for his confidence and sponsorship when Kelly and I were just starting out five years ago.

I am grateful to my three dear friends, Scott Lurie, a Podiatrist, Jeff Giller, a Periodontist, and Mark Meller, an Attorney/Entrepreneur, for helping me keep "all ends" covered when they listen and advise me as I emote my ideas during rounds of golf and various sporting and social events. They epitomize the definition of friendship.

Lastly, every professional should have mentors and coaches. It works in sports, politics and business. I have been fortunate during my career to work with some of the best coaches in the field of dentistry. In particular, though, I would like to thank Drs. Rich and Dave Madow, Dr. Woody Oakes, Cathy Jameson, Dr. Roger Levin, Dr. Mark Hyman and, especially, Kirk Behrendt, for their encouragement and guidance in developing my wonderful new career. Kirk had a major role in convincing me to pursue my vision of "Making a Difference in Peoples' Lives." I see the difference that I have made in the practices and lives of some of the dentists and team members that I have worked with and I am grateful to have this opportunity.

Section Five:

About the Author

B etween 1999 and 2002, Dr. Katz was out of work on disability and had virtually lost his practice to a series of life tragedies. Tapping into years of attending Practice Management courses, he embarked on establishing a clear Vision of the Practice he wanted to develop. He surrounded himself with a great team, trained them well and implemented systems that enabled the team and Dr. Katz to build a multi-million dollar practice out of the ashes. He is the senior Partner in Smiles On Broadway Dental Care in Malverne, NY. He is a graduate of Columbia University and the Washington University School of Dental Medicine. He has achieved Mastership in the Academy of General Dentistry and Fellowship in the International College of Dentists. He is an attending at North Shore University Hospital and has been the team Dentist for the New York Jets Football Team and a Dental Consultant for Fox News in New York.

As the founding Partner of Smile Potential Dental Practice Coaching, Dr. Katz enjoys sharing his secrets for success with dentists throughout the country through lecturing and one-on-one coaching with his partner in Smile Potential, Kelly Fox-Galvagni. He lives in Roslyn Heights, NY with his wife, Regina, an Eating Disorders Therapist, and he has three beautiful daughters Heather, Nicole and Allison, aged 18-26; proof, he says, that God has a sense of humor. He enjoys spending time with his family, playing golf and riding around with the top down on his convertible, regardless of the season.

Section Six:

About Smile Potential

D uring the early part of 2009 many dentists were starting to blame slowdowns in their practices on the crisis in our economy. It was during this period that Mitch Cutler and I sat down to discuss what other dentists were describing. Our practice was not experiencing the same phenomenon. My assumption was that the strategies that we had applied in our practice were a continuation of what we had done to recover from the situations that destroyed our practice several years earlier. Mitch thought that much of what we were doing could be helpful to practices trying to recover from their own, more recent, slowdowns. These discussions, and Mitch's encouragement motivated me to think about the idea of coaching other practices to help them reach their potential.

In the spring of 2009, when I told my team what I was planning to do, one of my clinical assistants introduced me to Kelly Fox-Galvagni, a former assisting colleague of hers from a previous practice. Kelly had a wealth of knowledge and also had a desire to help other dental professionals become better at what they do. Our first meeting, in April, 2009 clearly indicated that we were "on the same page" and that we were in total agreement on our philosophies for dental practice growth.

We delivered our first presentation, with encouragement from Mark Marinbach, on behalf of Nu-Life Long Island Dental Lab, at the Henry Schein facility in Woodbury, New York, in November, 2009. Since that time we have delivered over 100 presentations and we have spoken to over 5,000 dental professionals throughout the northeastern United States. Future presentations have us traveling across the US to work with dentists with shared concerns from other regions.

We have maintained a limited number of coaching clients, worked in around our "day jobs", as full-time practicing dental professionals. To date, we have worked with 35 dental practices in and around the New York metropolitan area. We have been thrilled to see these doctors SMILE from reaching their POTENTIAL.

A more recent development for Smile Potential has been working with some of the leading dental companies in training their sales representatives to improve the service that they provide to their dentist/clients by focusing on helping them grow their practices, instead of just selling their products. When practices grow from this information, the need for the practice to use more of these companies' products also increases and everyone wins. We are proud to work with Henry Schein, CareCredit, Straumann and Orapharma.

If you would like more information about Smile Potential, here is our contact information:

Smile Potential Dental Practice Coaching
116 Broadway – Malverne, NY 11565
Phone: 516-599-0214
Email: smilepotential@aol.com
Dr. Steven Katz – cell phone: 516-524-7573

Testimonials for Smile Potential

// In 2012 I had a well-established, 28 year old dental practice that seemed to be flat lining despite the high quality of service we provided. My team and I lacked enthusiasm and the practice had become stale. Our physical office reflected that. It was quite frustrating, but I really did not put much stock in the bold promises I'd seen advertised by practice management consultants.

None-the-less, two friends with similar practices cajoled me into attending a course given by Steve Katz and Kelly Fox-Galvagni. My friends promised me a day away from the doldrums of the office, lunch and some laughs. Besides, who wanted to take another implant course?

As I listened to their lecture, Steve and Kelly's sincerity, real life experience and practical approach clicked with me. Some of the things discussed seemed bold, but their genuineness swayed me and I scheduled a consultation.

Since enrolling with Smile Potential my practice has seen a 70% increase in production and a similar decrease in A/R. I now have a vibrant. enthusiastic team and that makes going to work everyday a joy.

Steve and Kelly put their hearts into working with a practice. Their knowledge, integrity, dedication and ability to motivate you, and your team is second to none. Professionally, hiring Smile Potential is the best thing I've ever done.

Thank you for bringing back the joy of dentistry!"

Steven M. Levy, D.M.D., Merrick, NY

"When I first heard Steve and Kelly speak at an event last year I was moved by their passion and the heart centeredness of their message. It spoke to me. I had been working hard on the development of my practice, we were being successful, though I felt there was still something missing...sitting in the audience that day it was clear.... what was missing was the positive culture that Steve and Kelly were modeling. With their guidance and intimate team coaching we have achieved it. Never in 30 years of practice do I remember having as much fun as I do today when I go into the office. I am part of a team that cares. We care for ourselves, each other, and our patients. Our patients are regularly telling us they feel it. And, we are consistently more productive and more profitable than ever. We just broke the million-dollar threshold for the first time in my 30 years of practice, up a little over 100 grand from last year. More important, we are having fun and getting great feedback from our patients. I am clear on my role as the leader of the practice. We have had some bumps in the road, and are

working quickly to confront and resolve conflicts that arise. We are a work in process. My vision has been realized and now I see new possibilities. We are setting up a fourth operatory with plans to bring on another hygienist... and down the road perhaps an associate/ partner/ successor."

Thank you Steven and Kelly".

Dr. David Lerner. Yorktown, NY

"I started my practice from scratch 5 years ago. Dental School taught me dentistry but left me unprepared for the business aspect of the practice. After struggling for four years I was determined to find a better way. I interviewed several practice management consultants and I came across Smile Potential.

Dr. Katz and Ms. Fox-Galvagni took a 360° view of my practice. They conducted training to identify and suggest ways to improve the practice right from day one. They walked us each step of the way to implement the systems that needed to be developed. Their expertise helped us increase our production and collection by 45% in one year. My staff and I absolutely loved working with them. My staff and I are very excited about going to work. We have a new energy in our practice.

Steven and Kelly are very approachable and hands on. Steven is a practicing dentist and Kelly is a D.A.N.B

Visiting

certified dental assistant. Substituting Smile Potential with someone who just has a business degree is like substituting a key ingredient in a recipe.

Smile Potential is based in Long Island. This makes it so much better compared to working with someone who is not local and is not familiar in dealing with the unique problems associated with practicing in Long Island. I strongly recommend Smile Potential. Call us for any questions.

Thanks Steve and Kelly!"

Dr. Monika Bhatia, Hicksville, NY

"In these hard times, my practice was stagnating. There was dissention among the staff. I knew that my business needed a boost. I decided to employ a local dental coaching team, Smile Potential. Immediately I saw results- there was a positive change in attitude among the staff and an increase in profits. Dr. Steven Katz's easy-going, informative approach to dental practice management and Kelly's ever-present upbeat attitude are a winning combination. I highly recommend them. You can bank on it!"

Anthony Falciano DDS, MAGD
Oceanside, New York

"I signed up with Smile Potential in December, 2010. Our monthly numbers were low; our new patient numbers were even lower.... I was under the misconception that if you were a great Dentist and truly cared about your work and patients everything else would fall into place. I was wrong. Since Steve and Kelly gave us direction, helped us establish systems and pointed us in the right direction my practice has reached a new level. It has been a lot of work and having the right staff in place is crucial. It continues to be a challenge to stay the course but Steve and Kelly have supported us whenever I need them. I highly recommend Smile Potential to any practice that feels they can be doing better. It has made practicing Dentistry go so much smoother, and my team enjoys the challenge and their role in our practice."

Dr. Nicholas Laudati, Smithtown New York

"I thought that after being in my practice for 35 years that decreases in productivity and growth was normal. I blamed the economy. I developed an accepting attitude and hoped for a miracle.

Instead of letting everything stagnate I hired Smile Potential to regenerate my practice and my thinking. They have succeeded beyond my greatest hope. Steve and Kelly have brought enthusiasm and joy into my practice. My staff and I feel empowered by the changes they suggested.

No one was more skeptical than I was. Our Production tripled in six months and our collections followed. They have turned a morbid practice into a vital and exciting place to work."

Dr. J S, General Dentist, Eastern Suffolk, NY

"In my thirty plus years of private practice and teaching, I've come across most of the practice management gurus, consultants, and courses, none of which has helped me more or impressed me as much as Dr. Steve Katz. The greatest, single impact Dr. Katz has had on my practice and me is his ability to identify the positives of my practice and make it better.

I was a mentor to Steve over 20 years ago when he was in his residency. Now, he has returned the favor, by instilling in me simple concepts, systems and principals, which enabled me to retire early and comfortably. Thank you Steve!"

Dr. Fred Danziger, Charleston, SC

"I have attended countless seminars. They always seemed to have the same advice, and a cookie-cutter mentality. Most suggestions just don't fit our practice.

242

Kelly really listened and understood our concerns. She has consistently given me practical systems and strategies that are easy to apply. I never imagined having a practice management consultant tailor a program for our practice. The results have been spectacular! With the knowledge and experience of Dr. Katz and Kelly, our staff is happier and much more efficient. Our collections are up, and our new patients have tripled. I recommend Smile Potential to any dental practice!"

Christine McGovern, Melville, NY

Office Manager

"Recently I had the opportunity to schedule a dental study club meeting with Dr. Steven Katz and Kelly Fox-Galvagni. Our group consisted of general dentists and specialists along with staff members.

It was a wonderful experience to hear the helpful suggestions that were presented by Steven and Kelly. Their insight into concepts that will work well in many offices was exceptional. I have never heard a more quiet room as they presented their material. It was a great learning experience and I suggest that you attend one of their lectures.

Thank you Steven and Kelly."

David M. Berk, DDS, MAGD, Woodbury, NY